The Strange and CURIOUS CASE of THE WACKY KID Health Questions

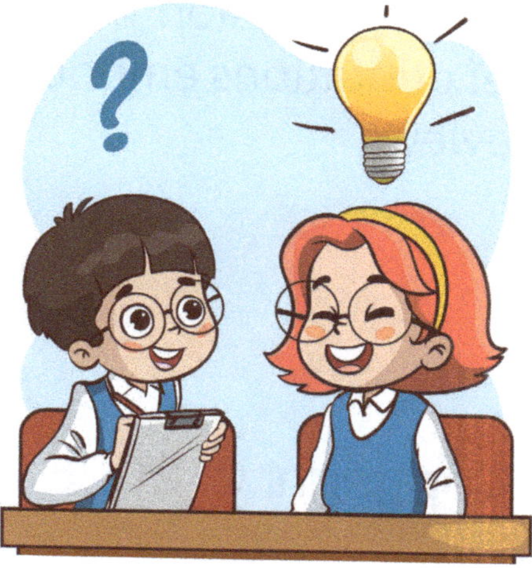

By Tony R. Wright

Dedication to children

"For my kids, Azariah and Antonia, whose laughter is my favorite sound"

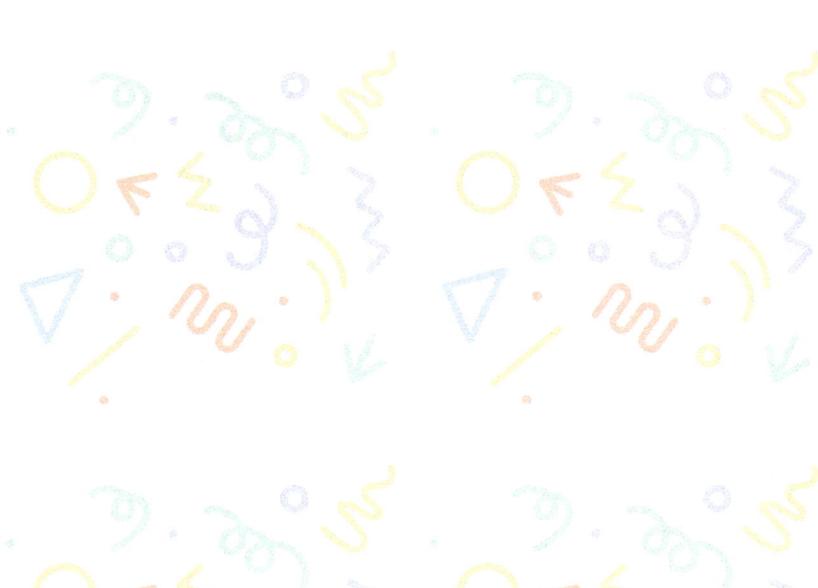

Introduction

Have you ever wondered how your heart beats, what happens to the food we eat, or why you do you sneeze? The human body is like a giant puzzle full of fascinating pieces working together daily to help you grow, play, and explore the world around you. It's no surprise that kids have so many questions about their bodies—after all, your body is your very own superpower!

This book is here to help answer some of the most common (and fun!) questions kids have about how our bodies work. Why do we need bones? How do we taste ice cream? Why do we yawn when we're sleepy? Whether you're curious about your brain, your muscles, or even why you get hiccups, you'll find easy-to-understand answers that make learning about your body exciting.

We'll take a journey through the amazing systems that keep you moving, thinking, and feeling every day. Along the way, you'll discover fun facts, like why your heart beats faster when you run, why your skin gets goosebumps, and why your belly button is a special little mark from when you were born. You'll also learn how to take care of your body, so it stays strong and healthy as you grow.

So, get ready to dive into YOUR incredible world! This book has fascinating questions and answers that will make you a human body expert in no time. Let's get started—you might be surprised at how awesome your body is!

CONTENTS

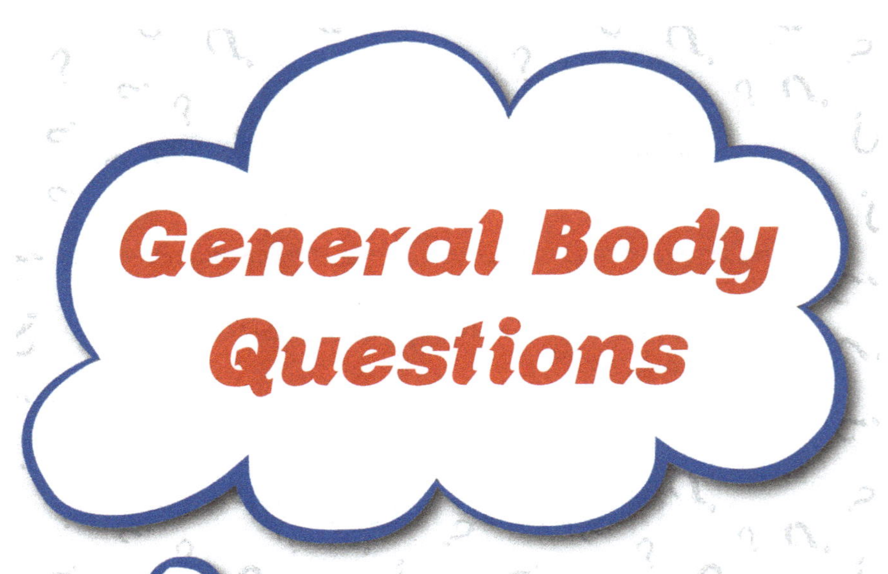

General Body
Questions

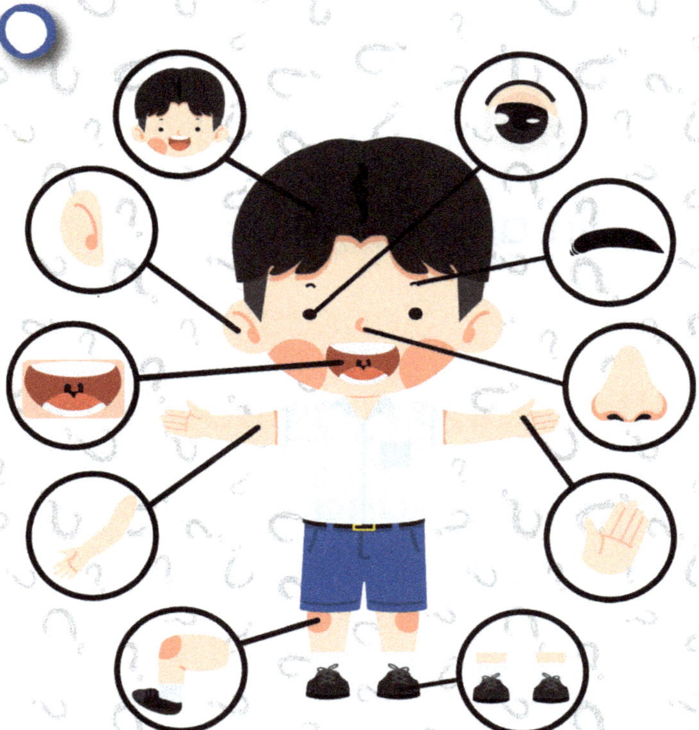

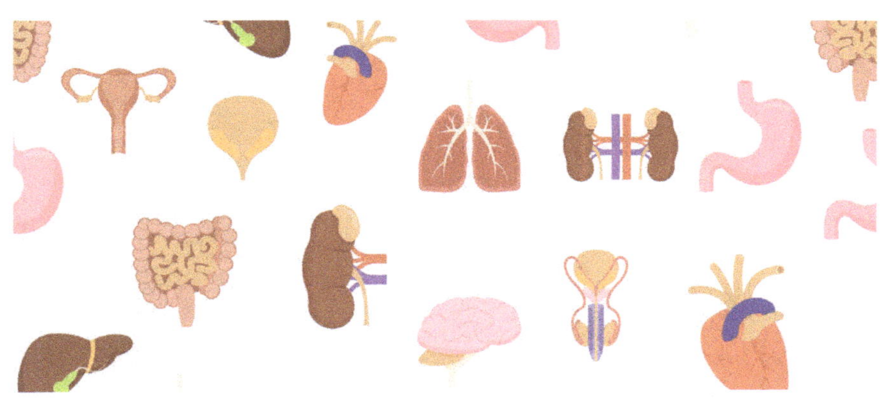

1. Why do we have a body?

Answer: Our body helps us move, think, grow, and stay alive.

2. What is the human body made of?

Answer: It's made of cells, tissues, organs, and bones working together.

3. How many bones do we have?

Answer: Adults have 206 bones, but babies are born with about 300.

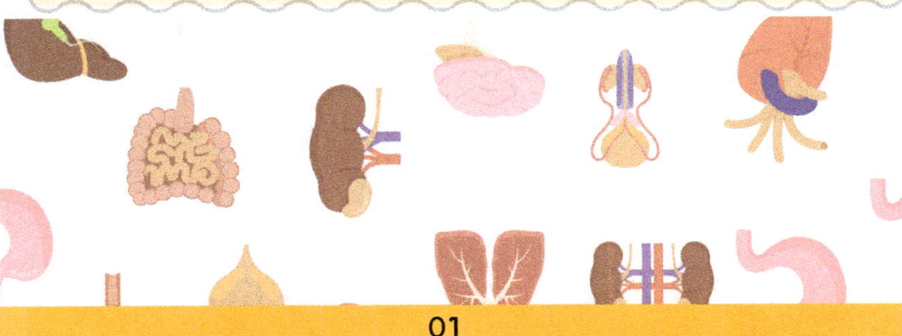

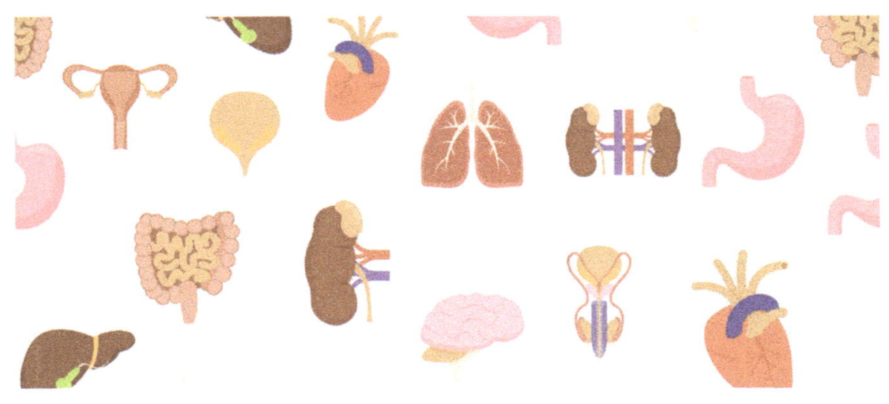

4. What are organs?

Answer: Organs are body parts like the heart, lungs, and brain that have important jobs.

5. What does the skeleton do?

Answer: It supports our body, protects organs, and helps us move.

6. Why do we need a brain?

Answer: The brain controls everything we think, feel, and do.

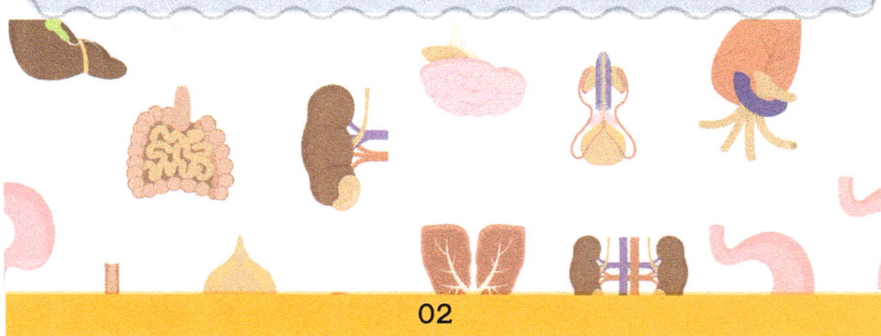

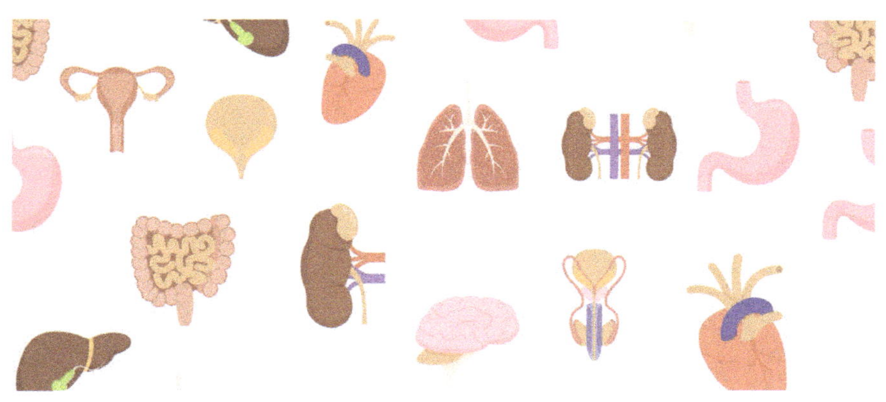

7. How does our body get energy?

Answer: We get energy from the food we eat.

8. How many muscles are in the body?

Answer: There are over 600 muscles in the body!

9. What are cells?

Answer: Cells are tiny building blocks that make up every part of our body.

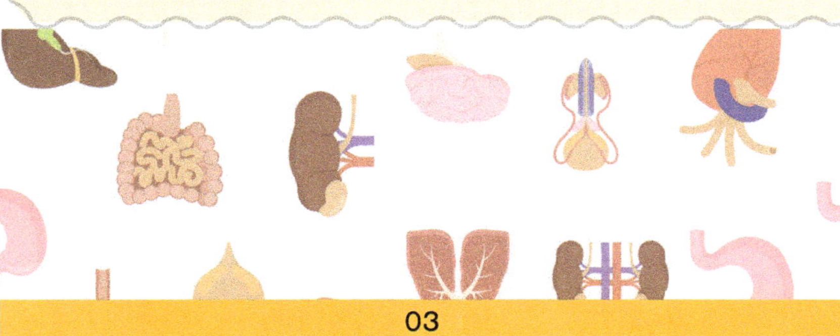

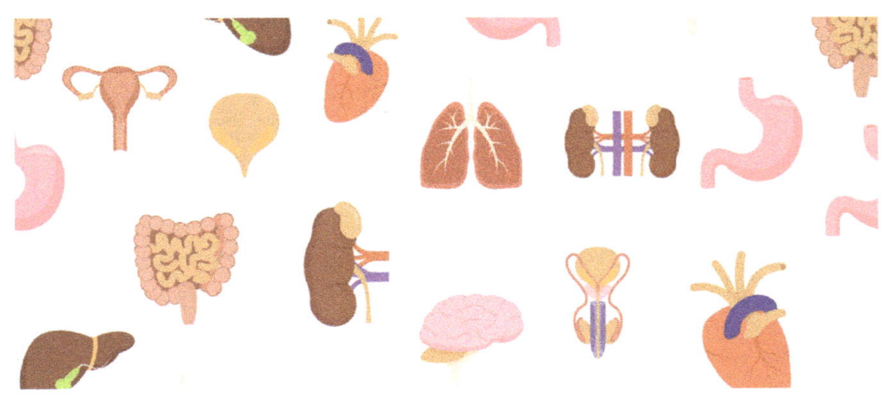

10. Why do we grow?

Answer: We grow because our bones and cells multiply as we age.

11. Why do we need food?

Answer: Food gives us energy and nutrients to stay healthy and grow.

12. What does the heart do?

Answer: The heart pumps blood throughout the body.

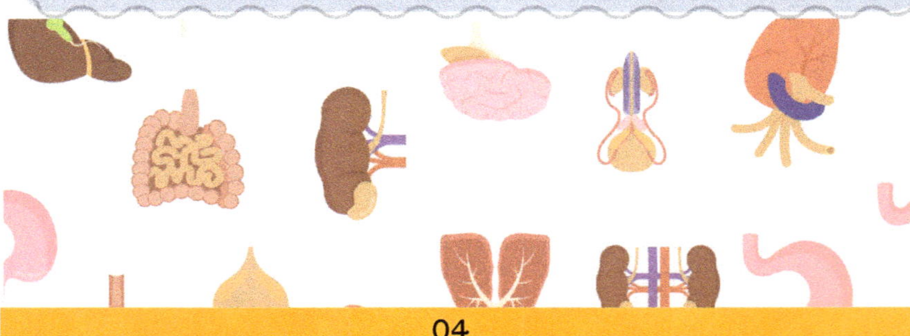

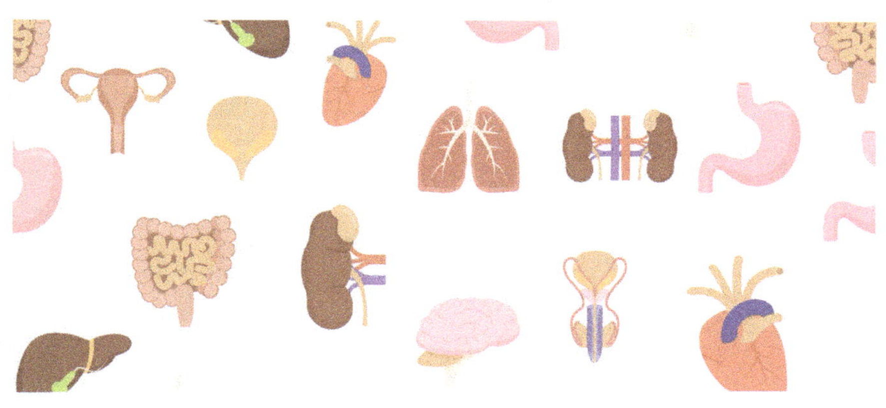

13. How does the brain send messages?

Answer: The brain sends messages through nerves.

14. How do bones heal after breaking?

Answer: Bones repair themselves by growing new tissue over the break.

15. What is the biggest organ in the body?

Answer: The skin is the body's largest organ.

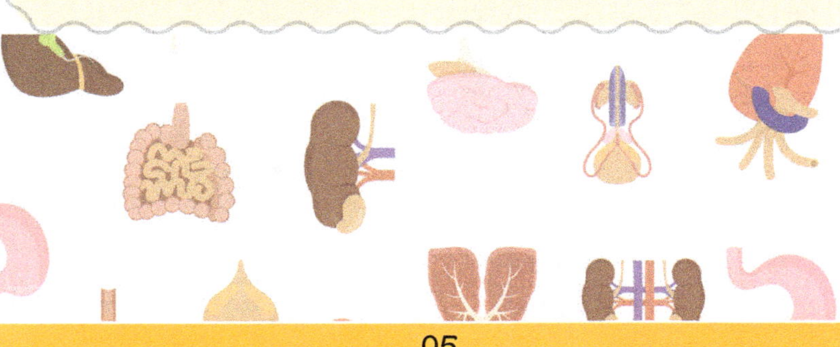

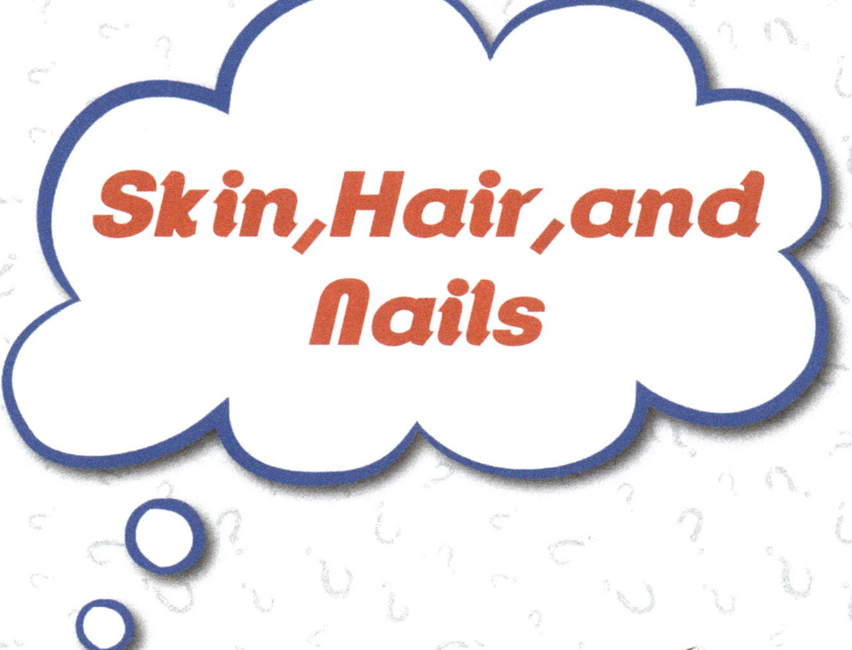

Skin, Hair, and Nails

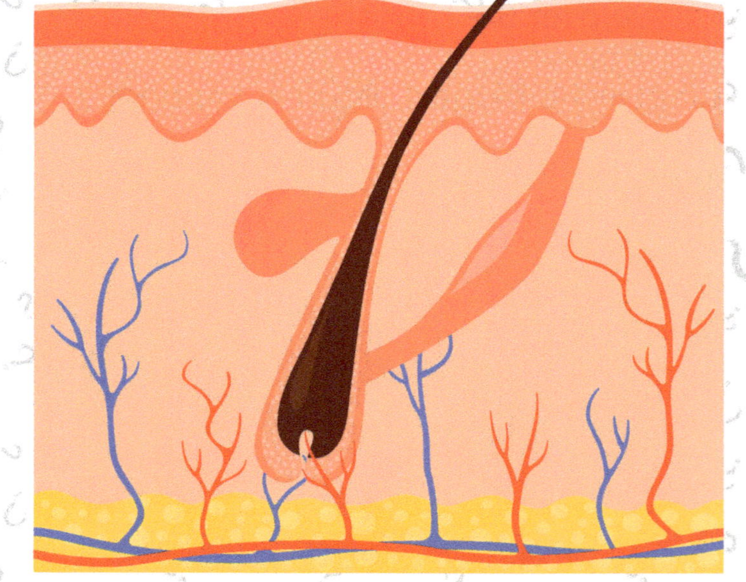

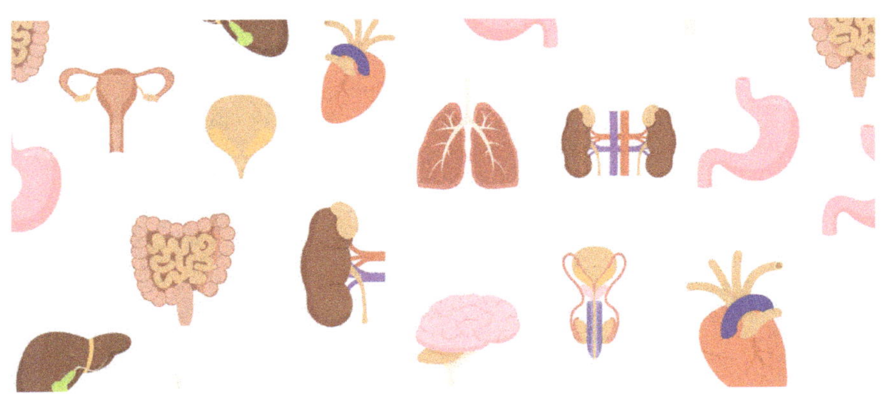

16. Why do we have skin?

Answer: Skin protects our insides and keeps germs out.

17. What is melanin?

Answer: Melanin is a pigment that gives skin, hair, and eyes their color.

18. Why do we have hair?

Answer: Hair keeps us warm and protects our skin.

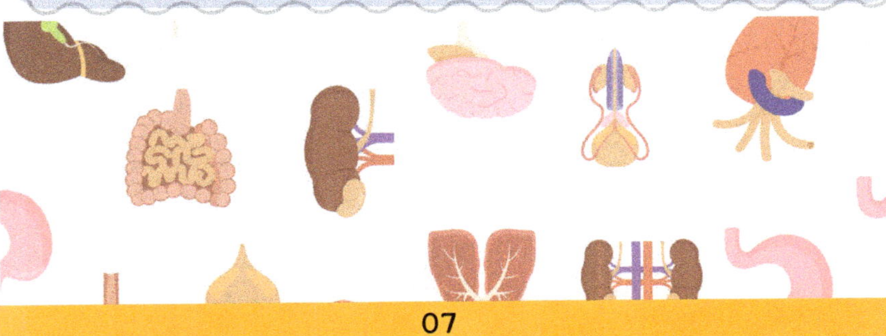

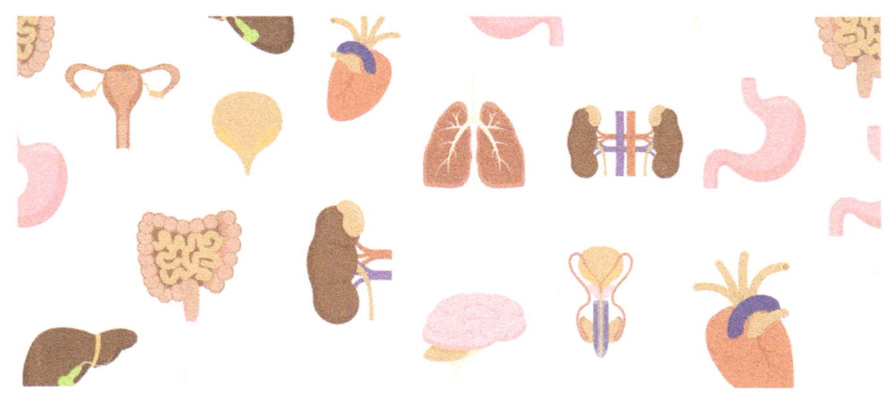

19. Why do we have fingernails?

Answer: Fingernails protect our fingertips and help us pick up small objects.

20. Why does our hair turn gray?

Answer: Hair loses its pigment as we get older.

21. What causes freckles?

Answer: Freckles are small skin spots with extra melanin caused by sunlight.

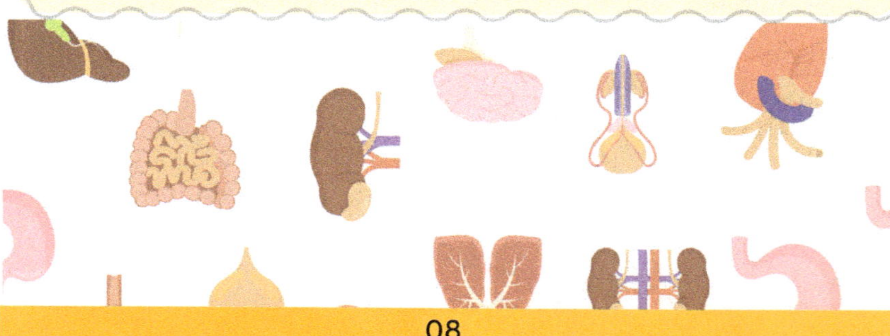

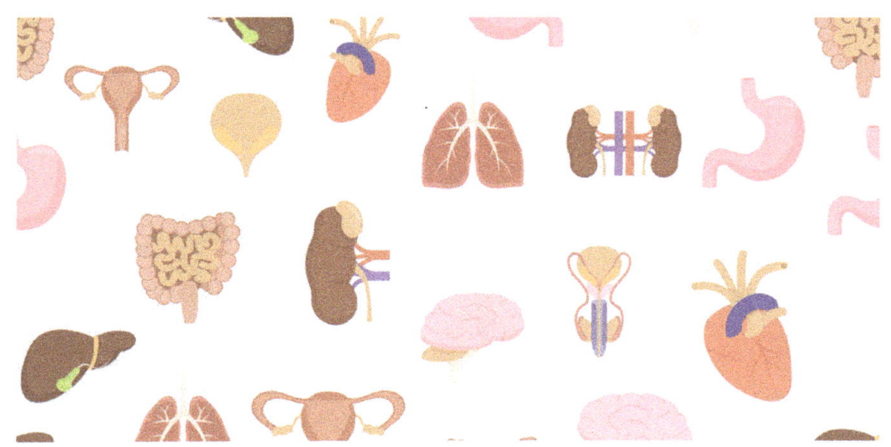

22. Why do we get goosebumps?

Answer: Goosebumps happen when tiny muscles in the skin tighten to keep us warm.

23. Why does skin wrinkle in water?

Answer: Wrinkling helps us grip slippery objects better.

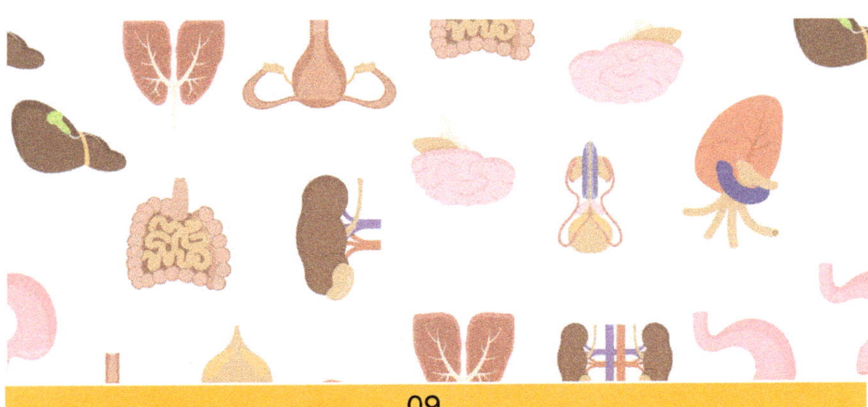

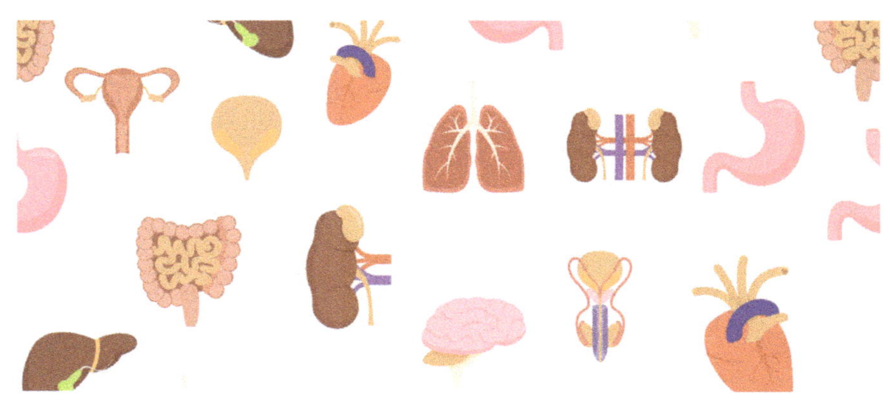

24. What are fingerprints for?

Answer: They help us grip things and are unique to each person.

25. Why do we itch?

Answer: Itching is caused by irritated skin or allergies.

26. Why do we sweat?

Answer: Sweating cools down our body when it's hot.

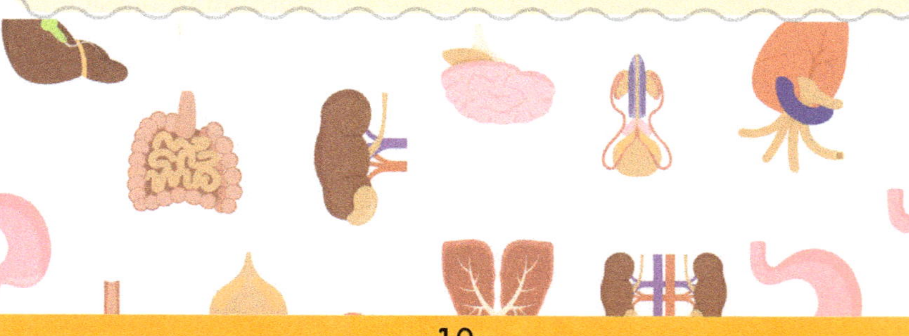

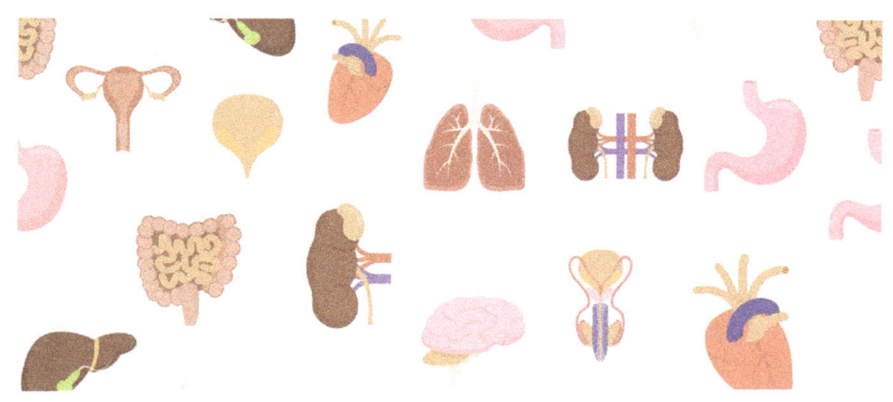

27. Why do bruises turn different colors?

Answer: Bruises change color as the body breaks down trapped blood.

28. Why do cuts hurt?

Answer: Cuts hurt because nerves in the skin send pain signals to the brain.

29. What is scar tissue?

Answer: Scar tissue forms when the skin heals from a deep cut or injury.

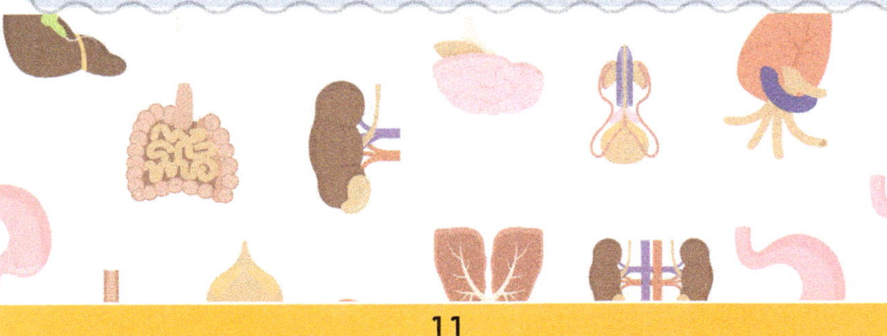

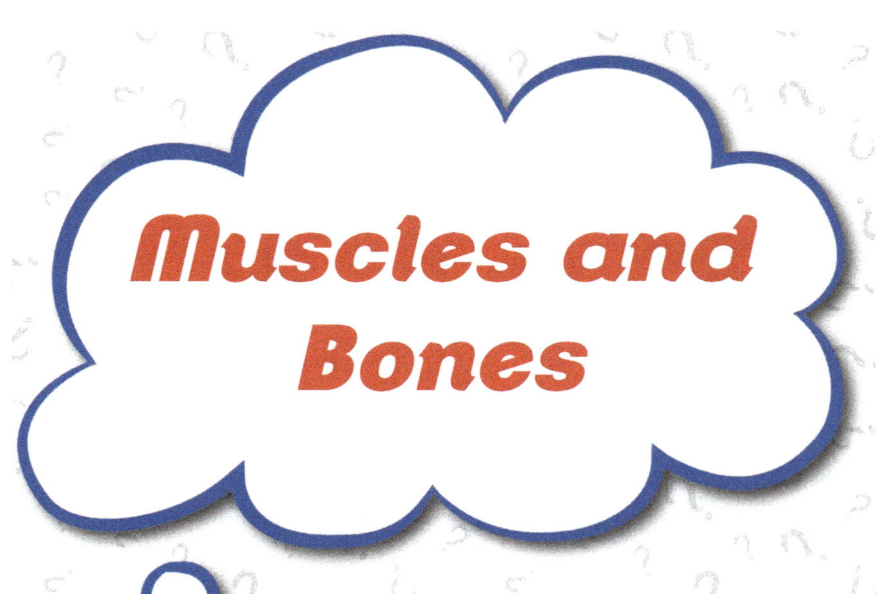
Muscles and Bones

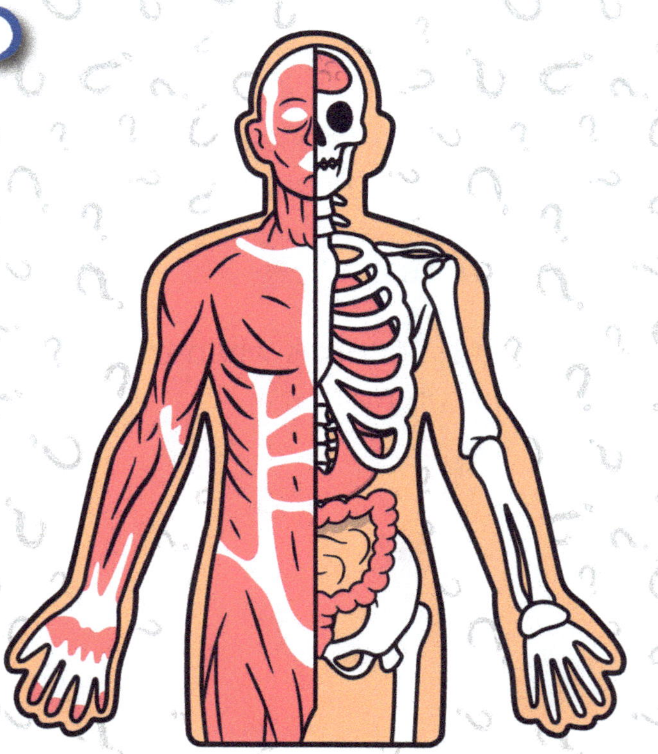

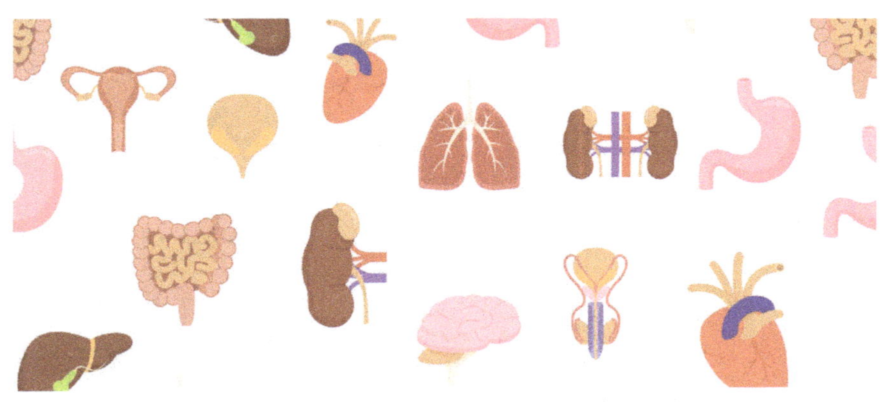

30. Why do we need muscles?

Answer: Muscles help us move, breathe, and even pump blood.

31. What is the strongest muscle?

Answer: The tongue is one of the strongest muscles for its size.

32. What is the biggest bone in the body?

Answer: The femur, or thigh bone.

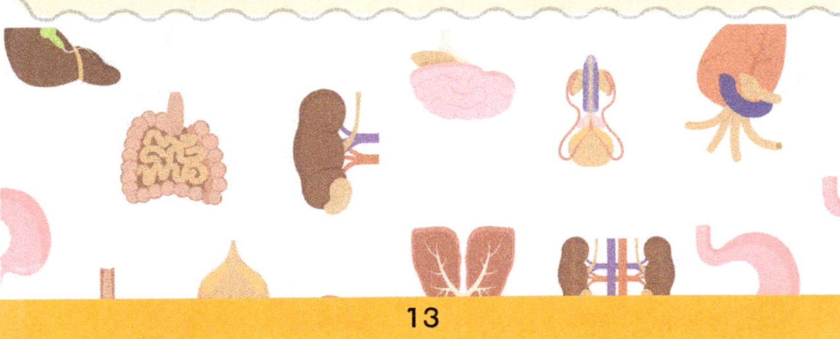

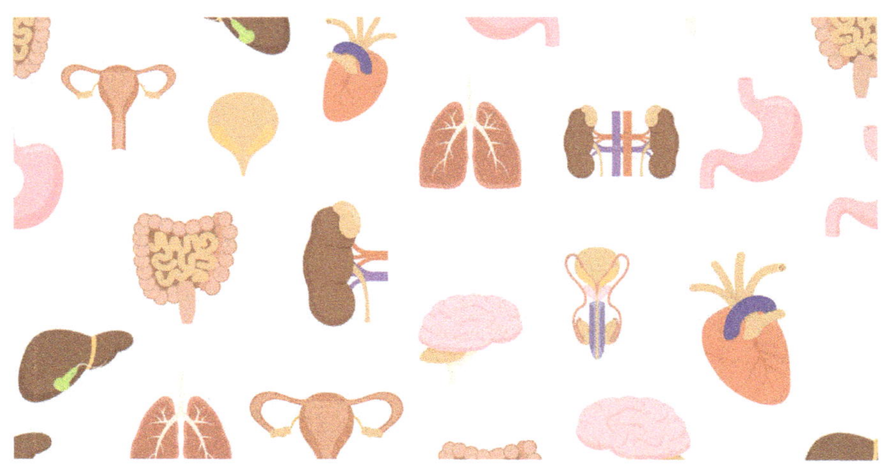

33. How do muscles grow stronger?

Answer: Exercising and eating healthy foods help muscles grow strong.

34. What happens when a muscle cramps?

Answer: A cramp is when a muscle tightens and won't relax.

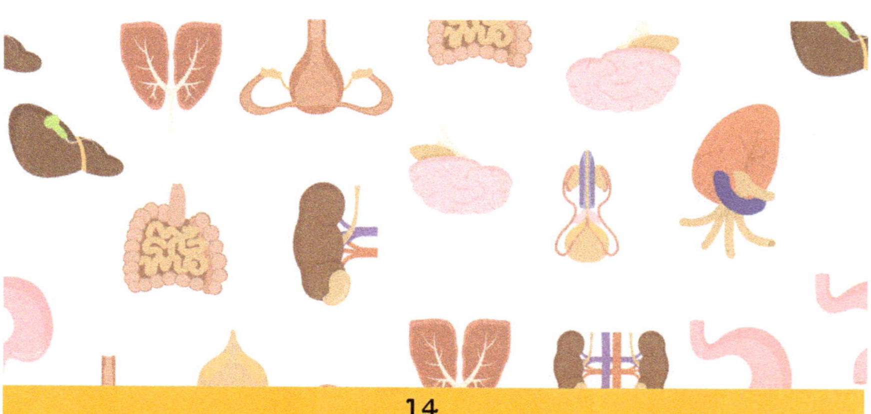

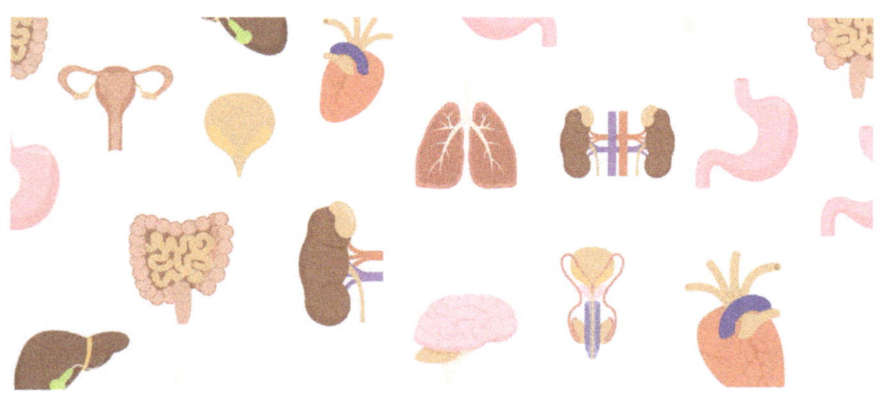

35. What is the smallest bone in the body?

Answer: The stapes, or stirrup bone, in the ear.

36. What is cartilage?

Answer: Cartilage is soft, flexible tissue that cushions joints.

37. Why do bones crack when we stretch?

Answer: It's from gas bubbles popping in the joints.

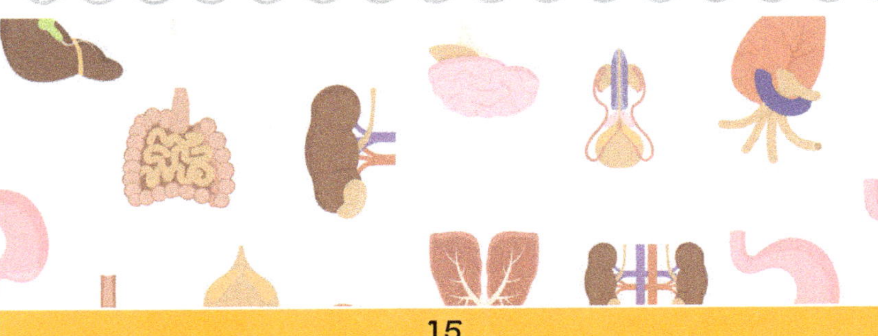

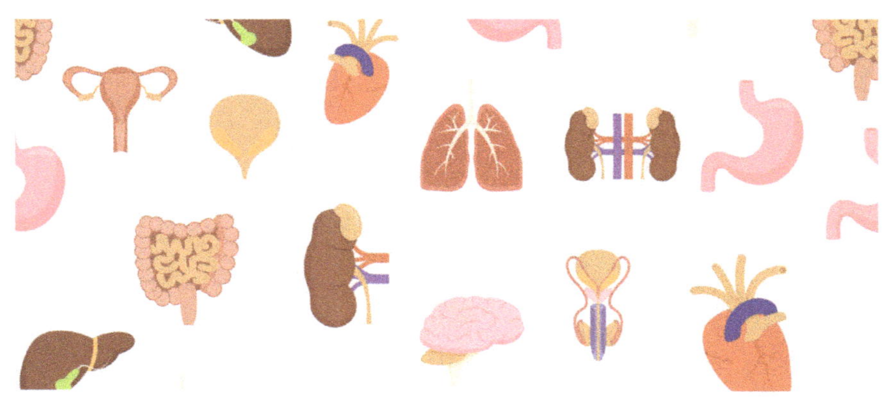

38. Why are bones white?

Answer: Bones appear white because they are made of minerals like calcium.

39. How does exercise help bones?

Answer: Exercise strengthens bones by keeping them dense and strong.

40. Why do we stretch?

Answer: Stretching keeps muscles flexible and ready for movement.

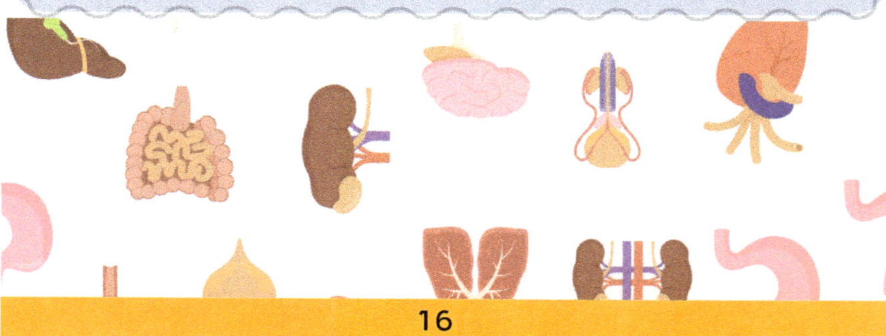

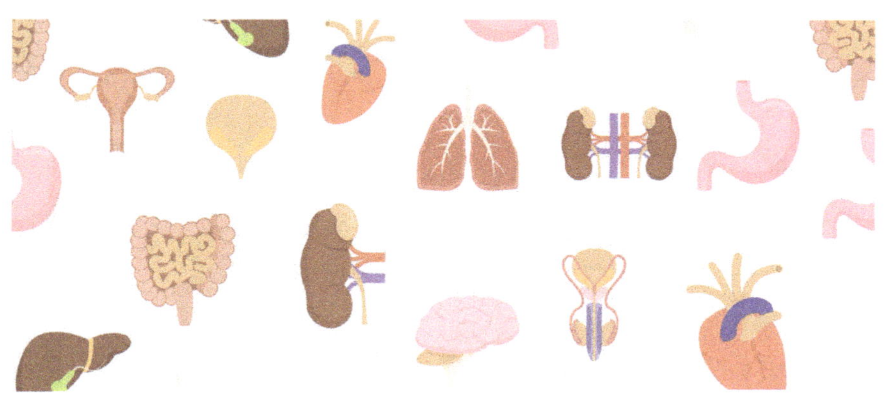

41. What are ligaments?

Answer: Ligaments are stretchy tissues that connect bones at joints.

42. Why are bones hard?

Answer: They contain minerals like calcium that make them strong.

43. What are tendons?

Answer: Tendons connect muscles to bones.

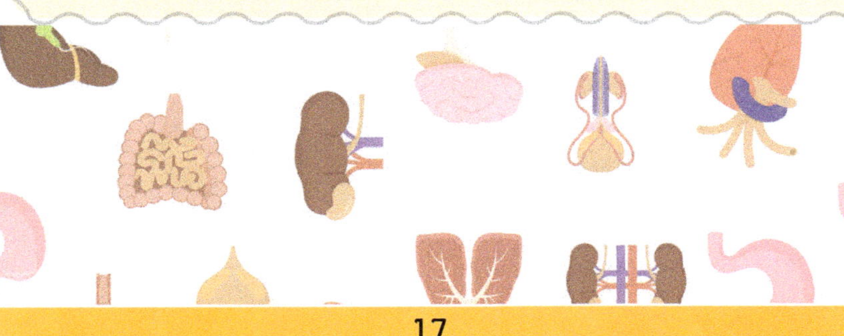

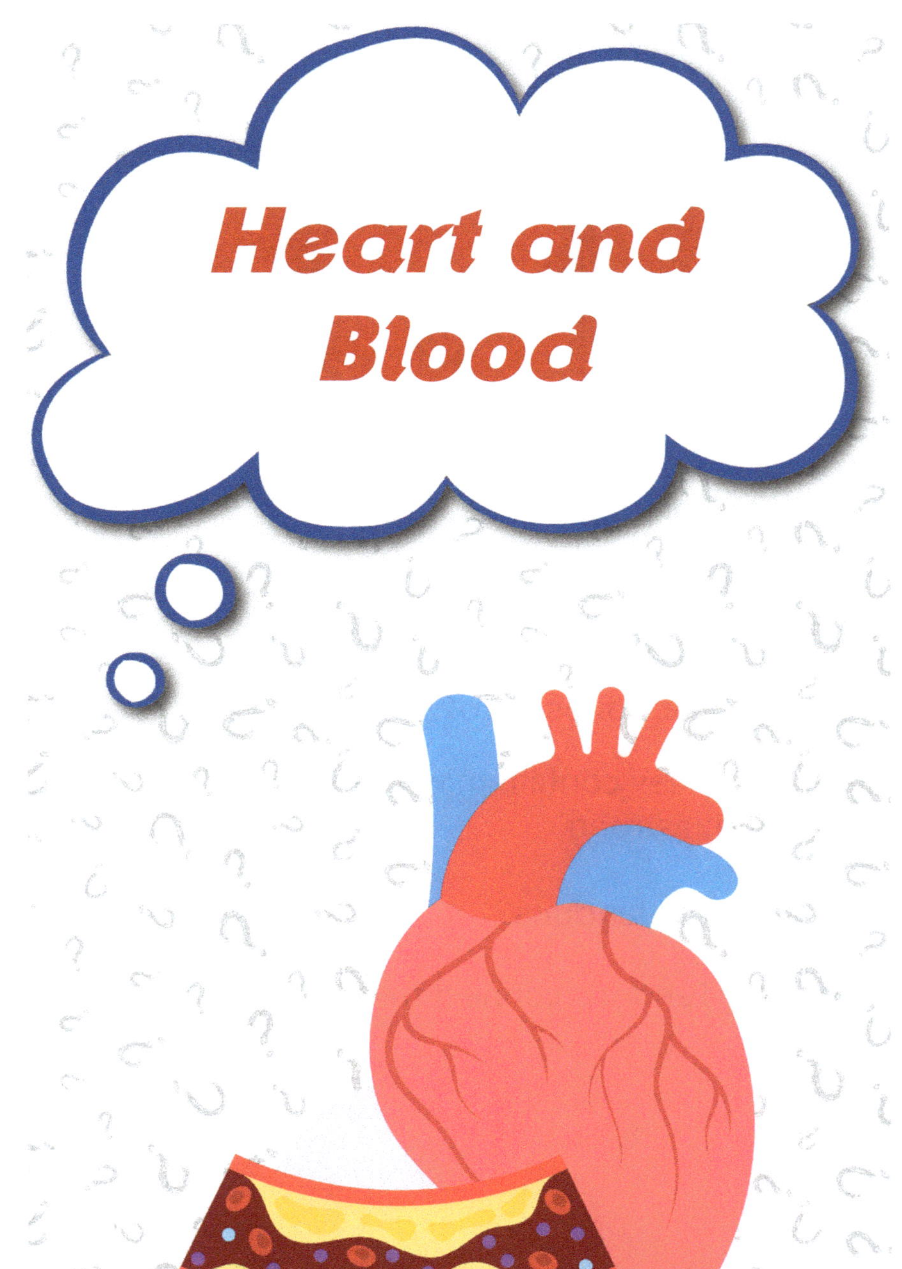

Heart and Blood

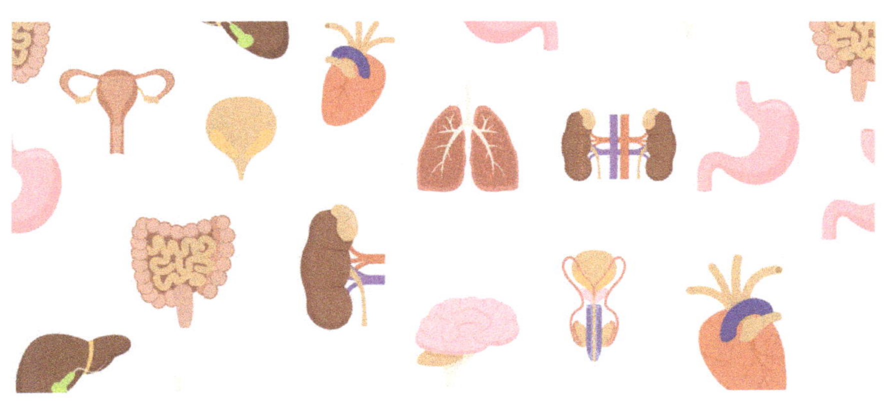

44. What does the heart do?

Answer: The heart pumps blood through our body.

45. How big is the heart?

Answer: It's about the size of your fist.

46. How many times does the heartbeat in a day?

Answer: About 100,000 times!

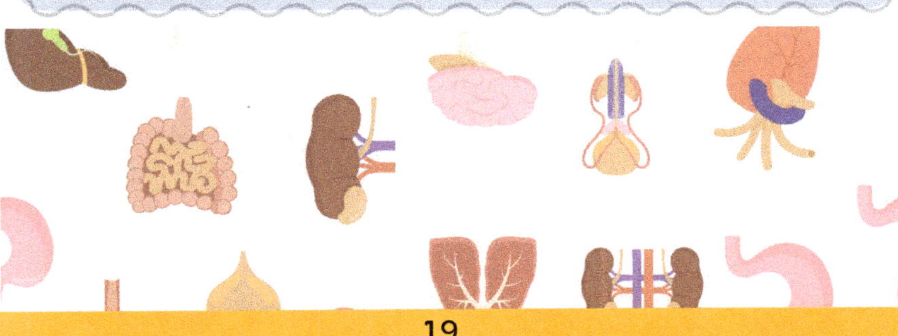

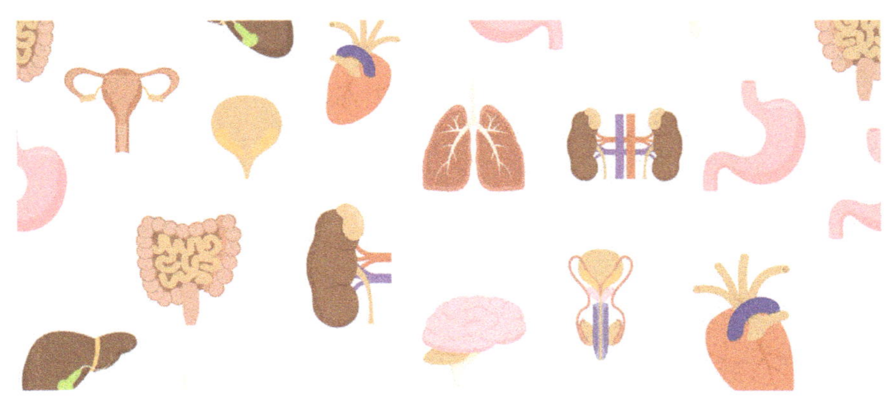

47. What is blood made of?

Answer: Blood has red and white blood cells, platelets, and plasma.

48. Why is blood red?

Answer: Blood is red because of a protein called hemoglobin in red blood cells.

49. What do red blood cells do?

Answer: They carry oxygen from the lungs to the rest of the body.

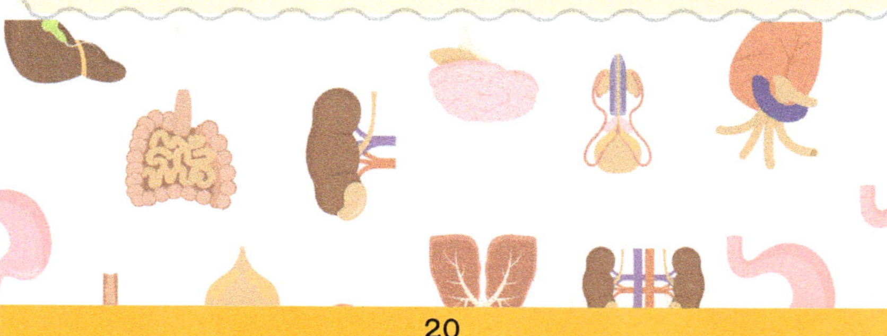

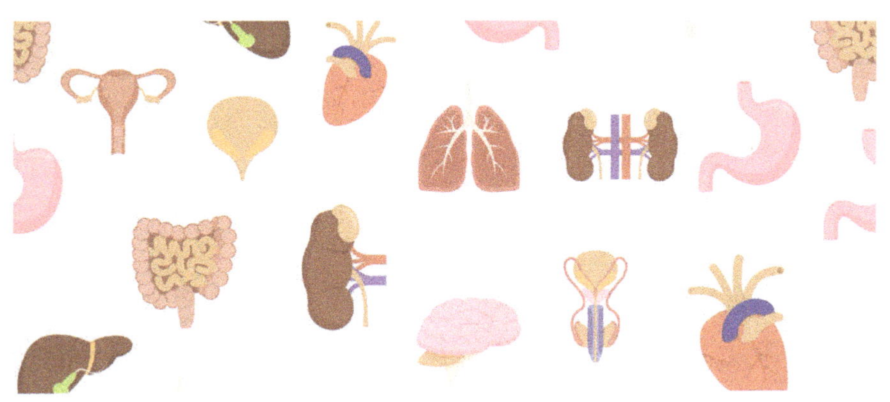

50. What do white blood cells do?

Answer: They fight germs and keep us healthy.

51. What are veins?

Answer: Veins carry blood back to the heart.

52. What are arteries?

Answer: Arteries carry blood away from the heart.

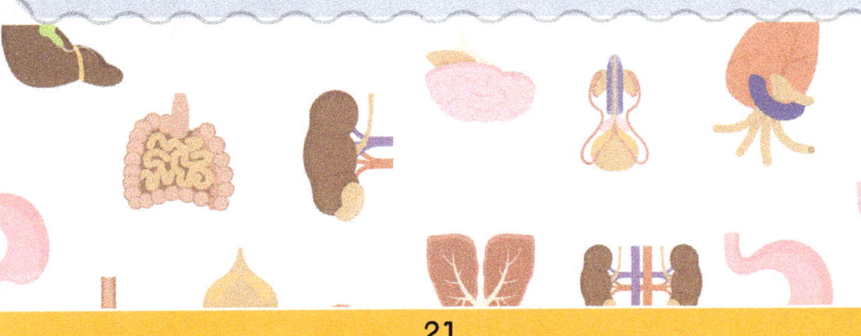

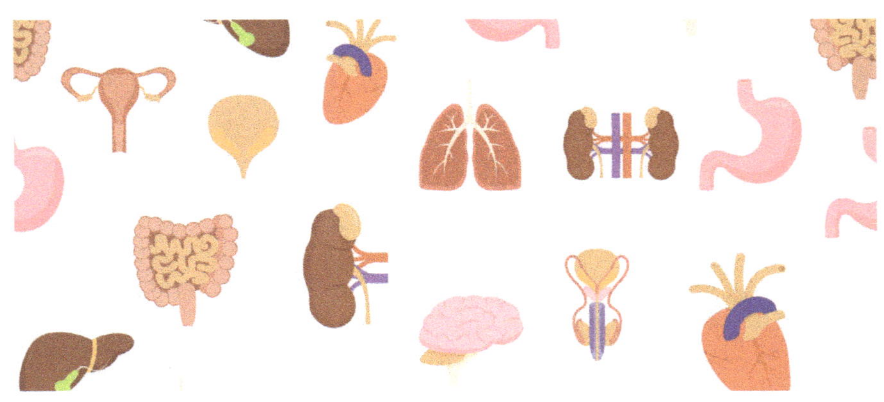

53. Why do we need blood?

Answer: Blood delivers oxygen and nutrients to our body and removes waste.

54. What is a heartbeat?

Answer: A heartbeat is the sound of the heart pumping blood.

55. Why do our hearts beat faster when we run?

Answer: Running makes the body need more oxygen, so the heart beats faster.

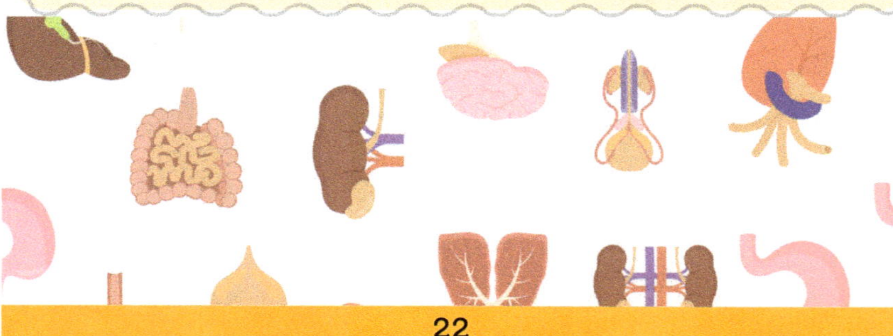

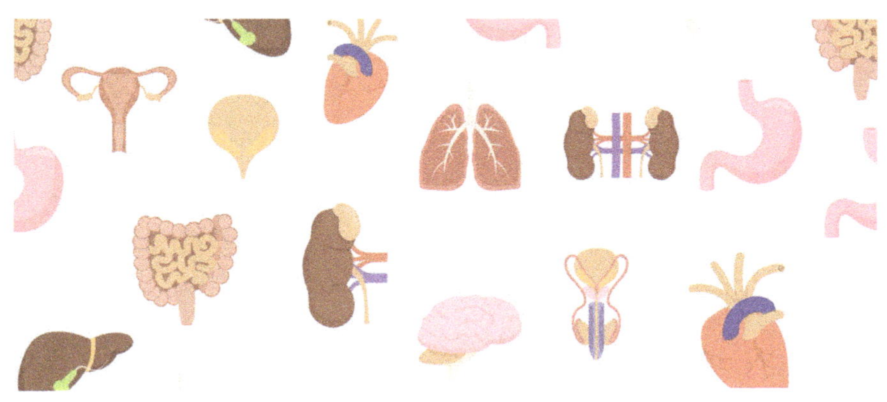

56. What is a pulse?

Answer: A pulse is the feeling of blood moving through an artery.

57. Why do we get bruises?

Answer: Bruises happen when small blood vessels break under the skin.

58. What is blood pressure?

Answer: Blood pressure measures how hard the heart pumps blood through the body.

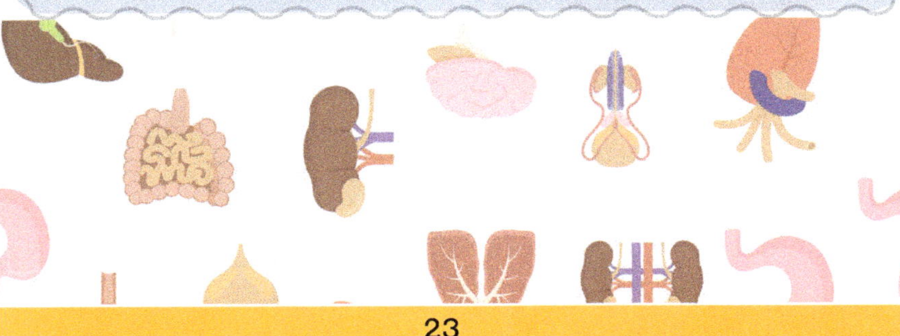

Lungs and Breathing

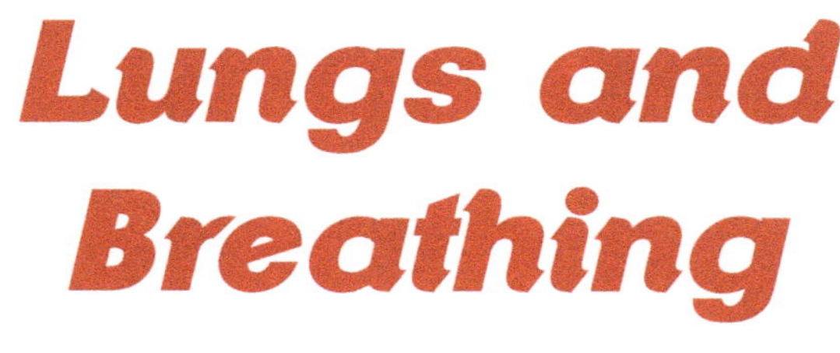

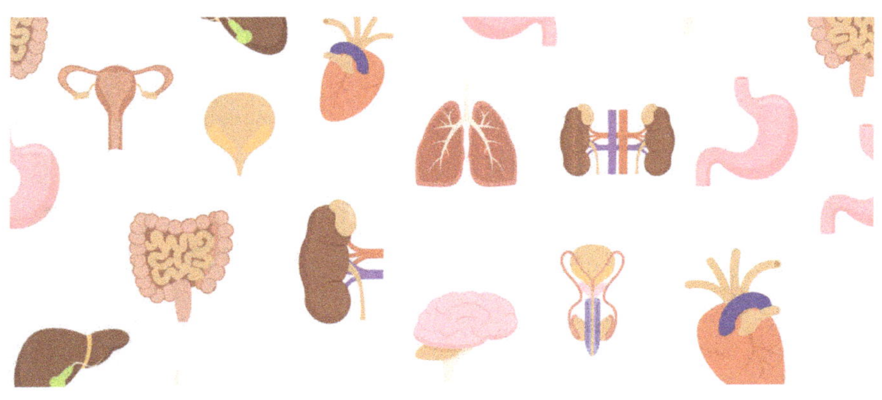

59. Why do we need to breathe?

Answer: Breathing brings oxygen into the body and removes carbon dioxide.

60. What are lungs?

Answer: Lungs are organs that help us breathe by taking in oxygen and releasing carbon dioxide.

61. How many lungs do we have?

Answer: Two – a right lung and a left lung.

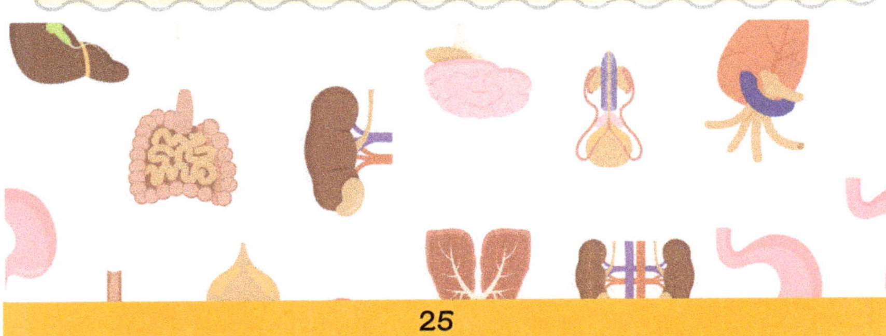

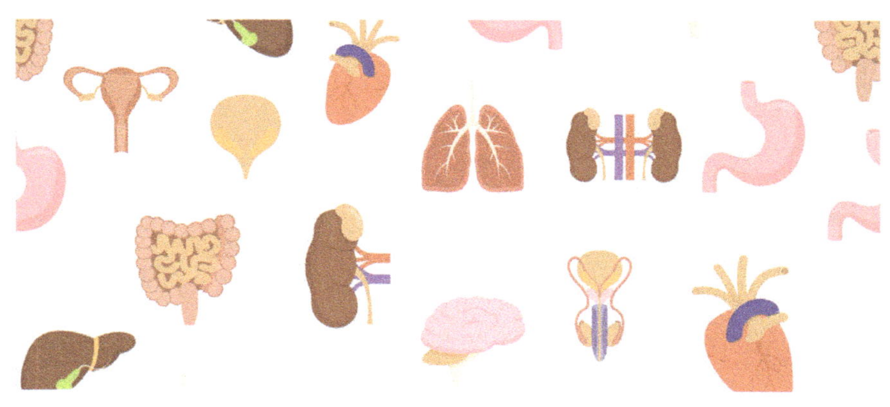

62. What happens when we inhale?

Answer: Air enters our lungs, bringing oxygen into our body.

63. What happens when we exhale?

Answer: We breathe out carbon dioxide, a waste gas.

64. Why do we yawn?

Answer: Yawning helps bring in more oxygen when we're tired.

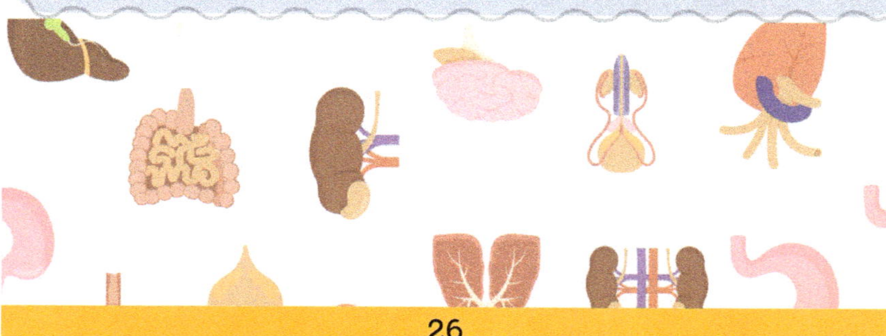

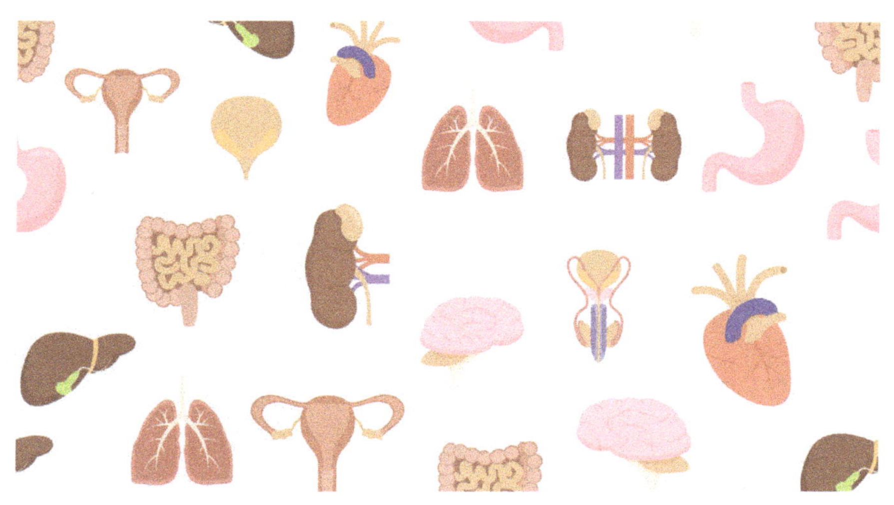

65. Why do we sneeze?

Answer: Sneezing clears irritants like dust from our nose.

66. Why does running make us breathe harder?

Answer: Running makes our body use more oxygen, so we breathe faster.

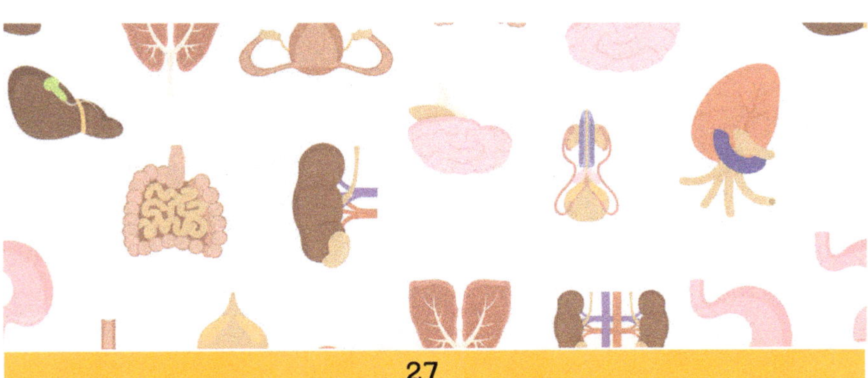

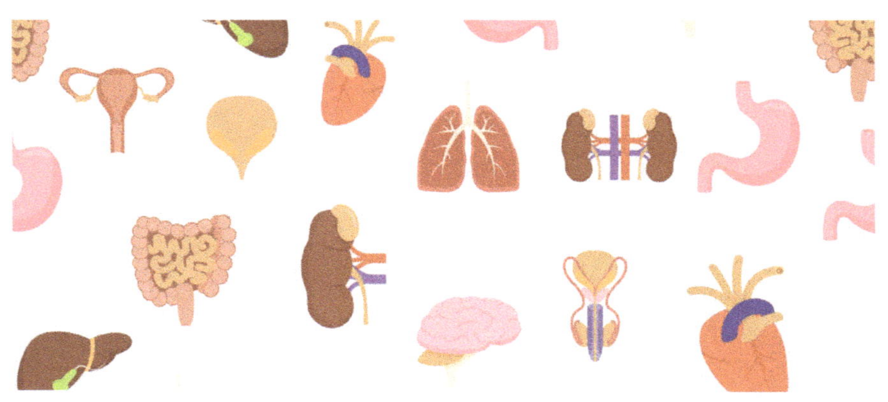

67. What is the diaphragm?

Answer: The diaphragm is a muscle that helps us breathe by moving up and down.

68. Why do we cough?

Answer: Coughing clears irritants from our lungs and throat.

69. What is mucus?

Answer: Mucus is a sticky substance in our nose and lungs that traps dirt and germs.

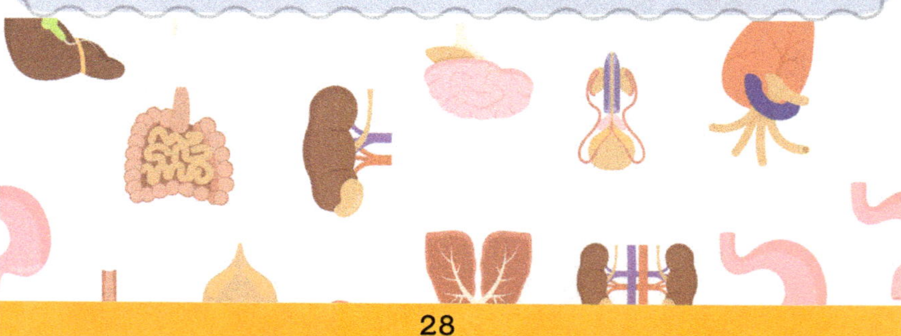

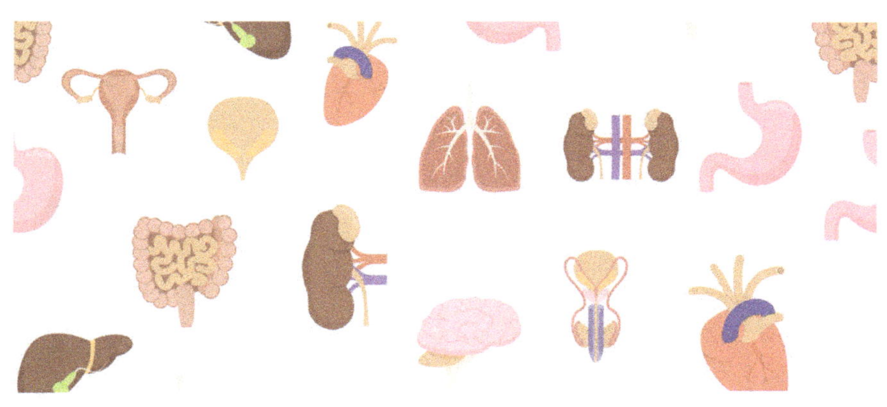

70. Why does cold air make us cough?

Answer: Cold air can irritate our throat and lungs.

71. What do tiny hairs in the nose do?

Answer: They filter dust and germs from the air we breathe.

72. How many breaths do we take each day?

Answer: We take about 20,000 breaths every day!

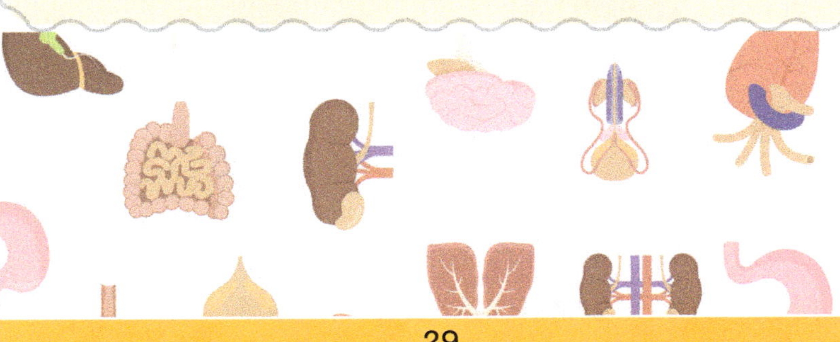

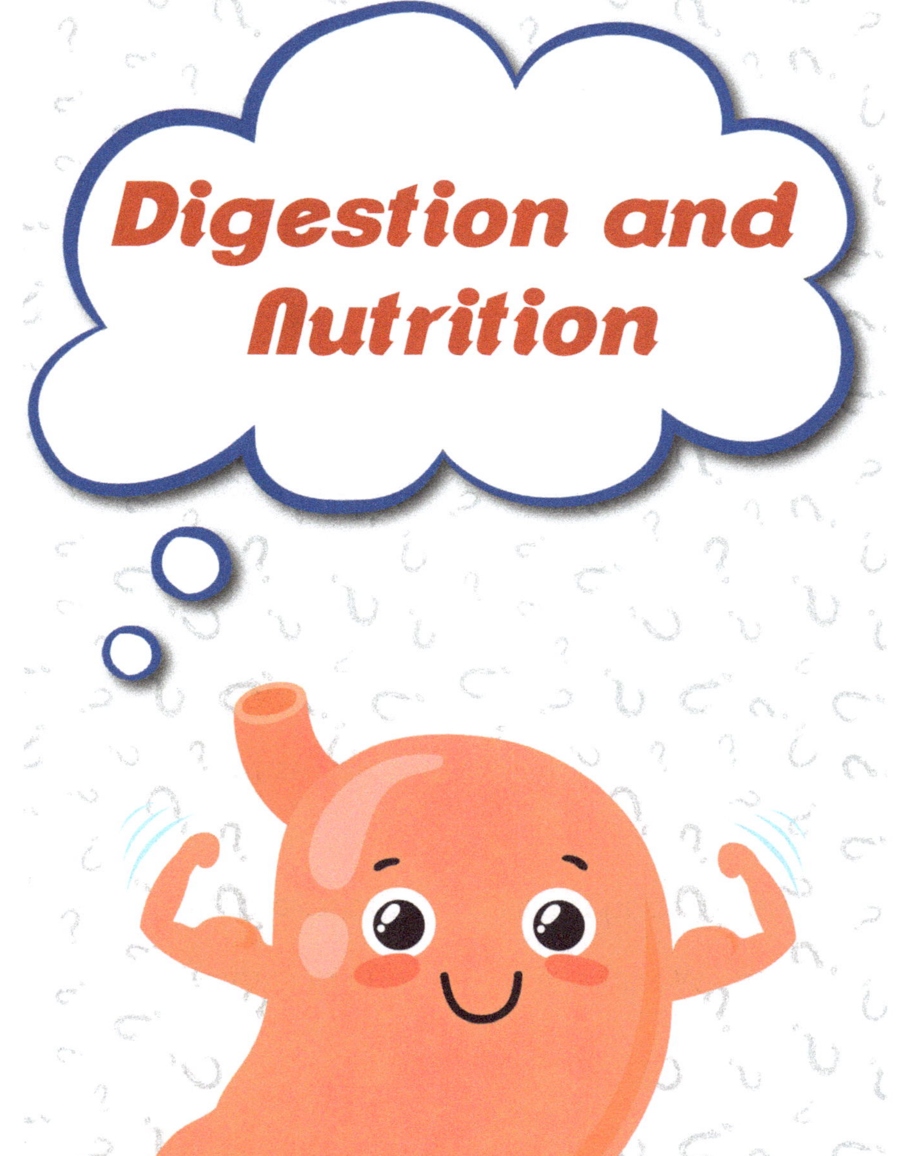

Digestion and Nutrition

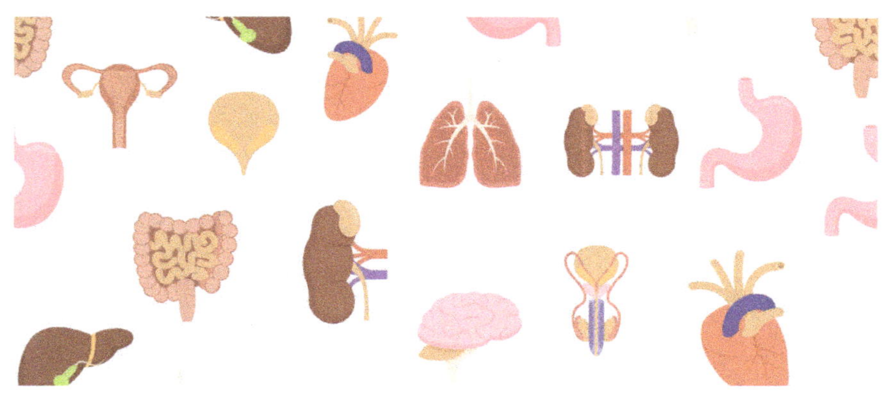

73. What happens to food when we eat it?

Answer: Food is broken down into nutrients that our body uses for energy.

74. What does the stomach do?

Answer: The stomach breaks down food with acid and enzymes.

75. What are intestines?

Answer: Intestines are long tubes where food is digested and nutrients are absorbed.

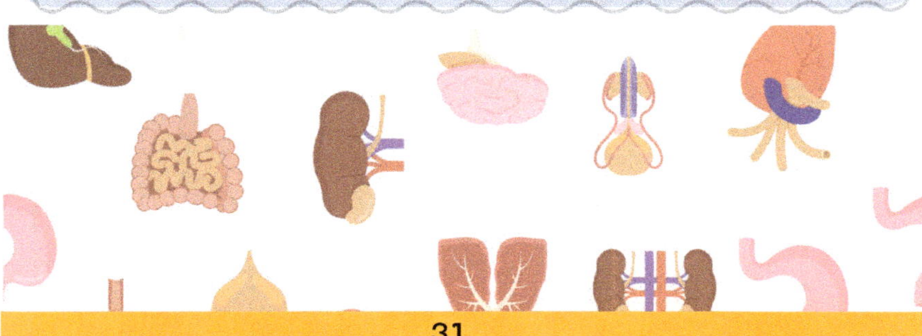

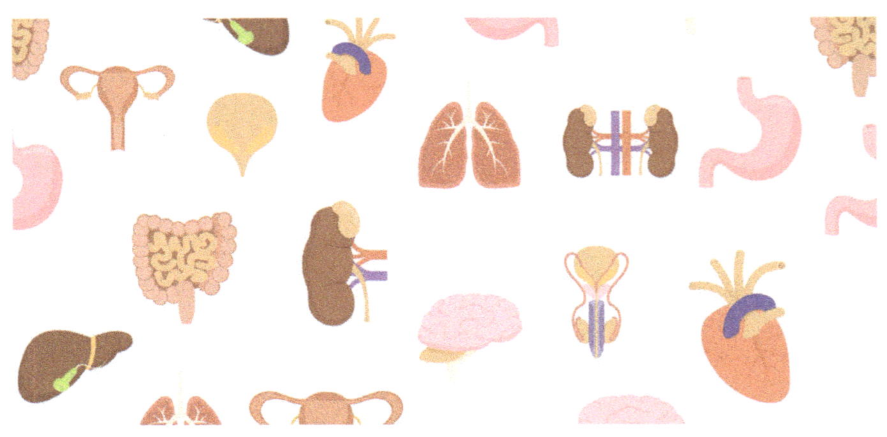

76. What does the small intestine do?

Answer: It absorbs nutrients from food.

77. What does the large intestine do?

Answer: It absorbs water and turns food waste into poop.

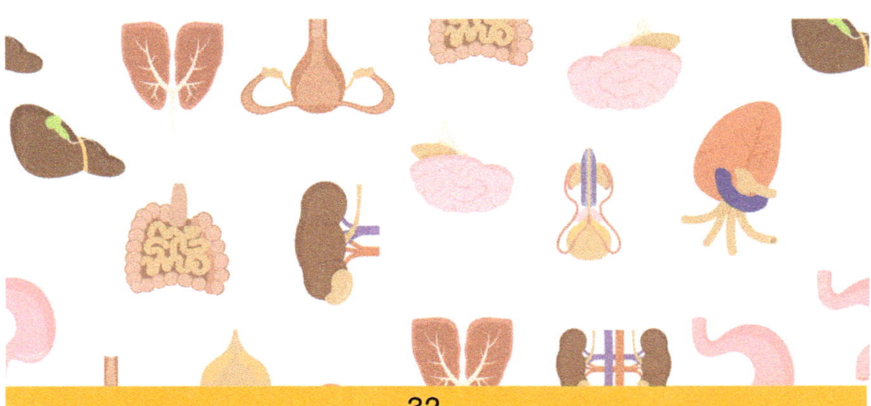

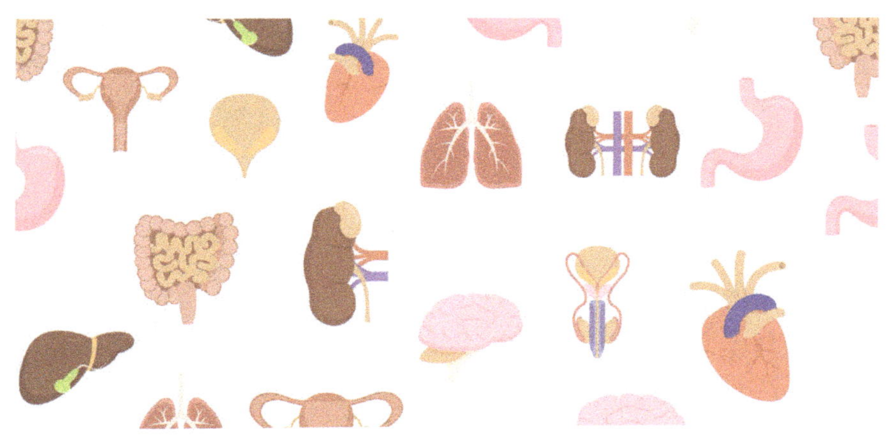

78. What is saliva?

Answer: Saliva is a liquid in the mouth that helps break down food.

79. Why do we get hungry?

Answer: Our brain signals hunger when the body needs more energy.

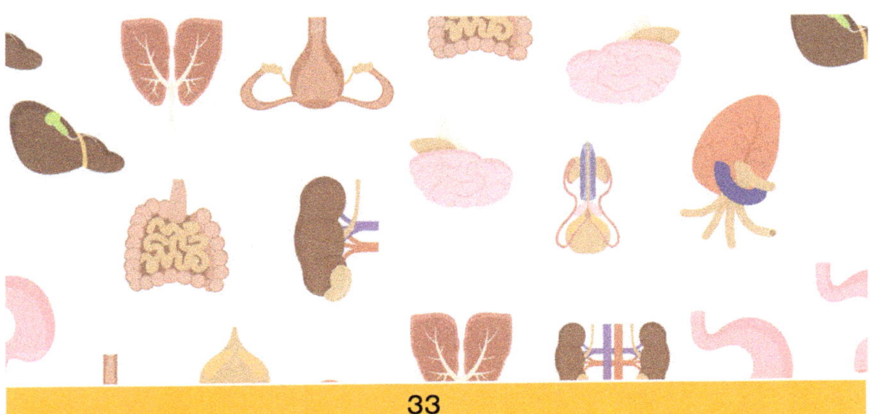

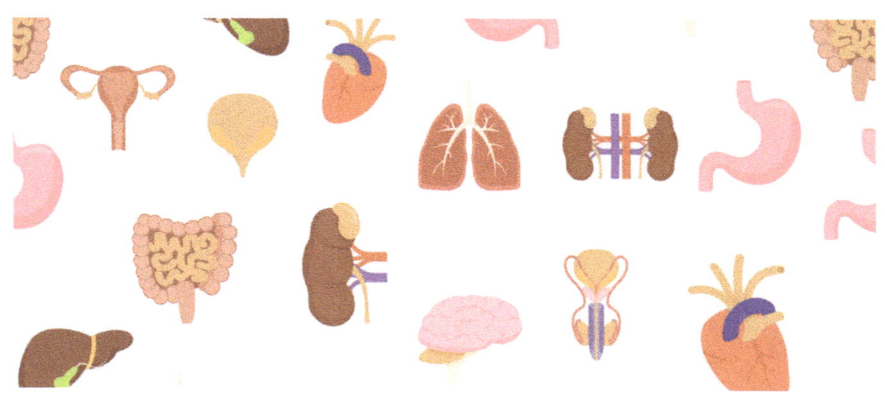

80. What is the liver's job?

Answer: The liver cleans the blood and helps digest food.

81. What is the pancreas?

Answer: The pancreas helps control blood sugar and make digestive enzymes.

82. Why do we need water?

Answer: Water keeps our bodies hydrated and helps digestion.

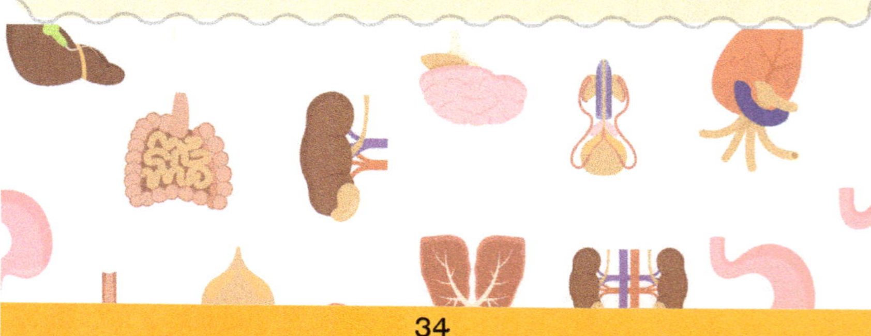

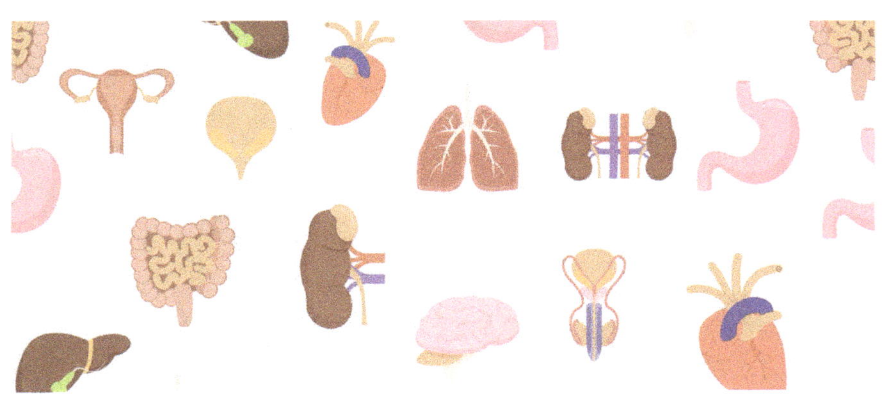

83. How long does it take to digest food?

Answer: It takes about 24 to 72 hours to fully digest food.

84. Why do we need fiber?

Answer: Fiber helps our digestion and keeps us regular.

85. Why do some foods give energy quickly?

Answer: Sugary foods break down fast, giving a quick energy boost.

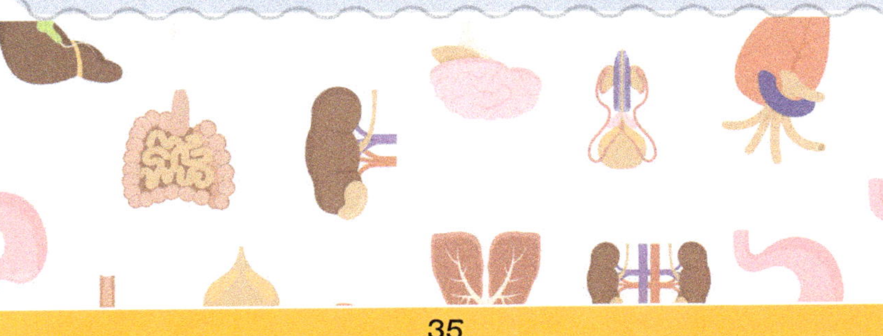

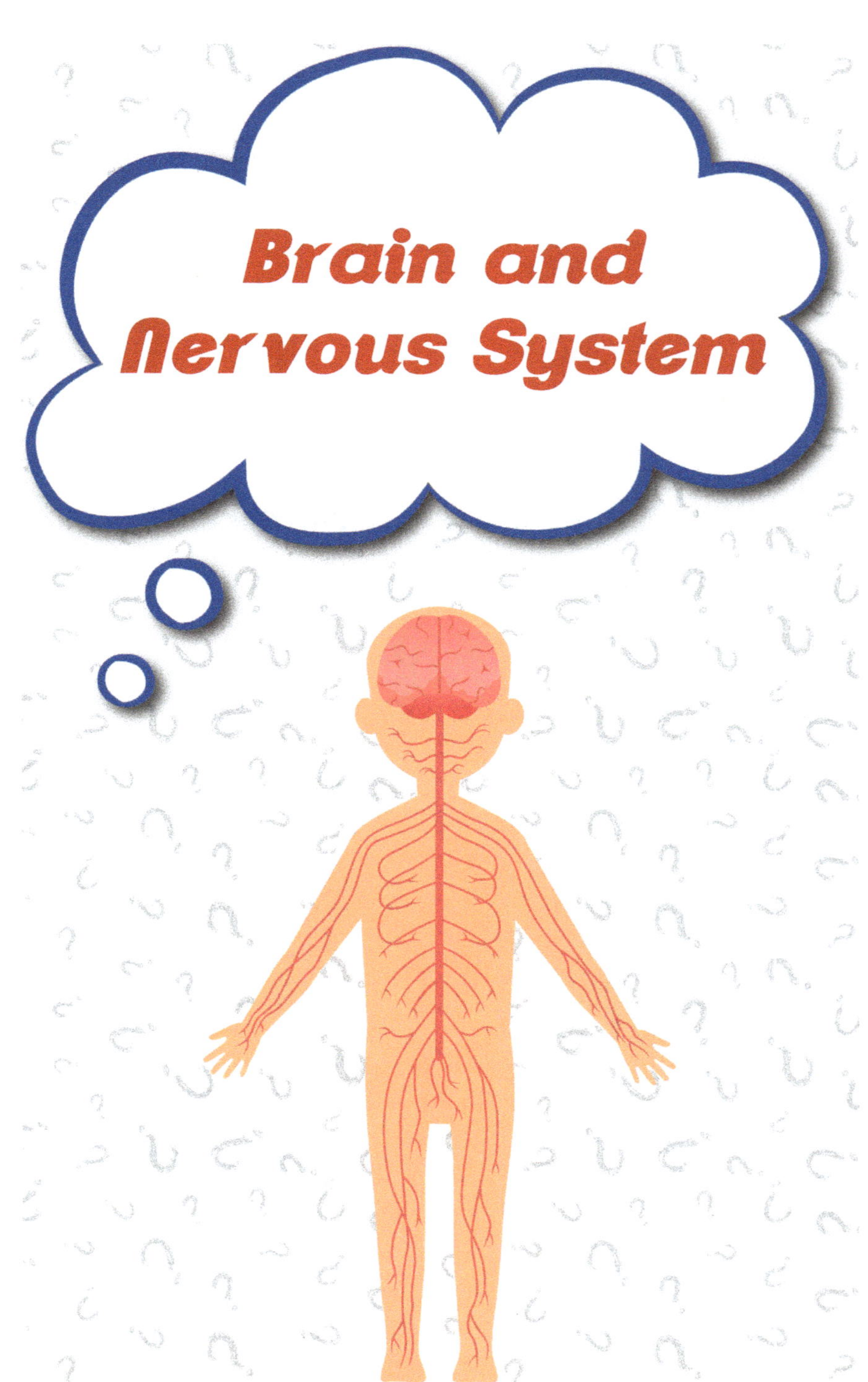

Brain and
Nervous System

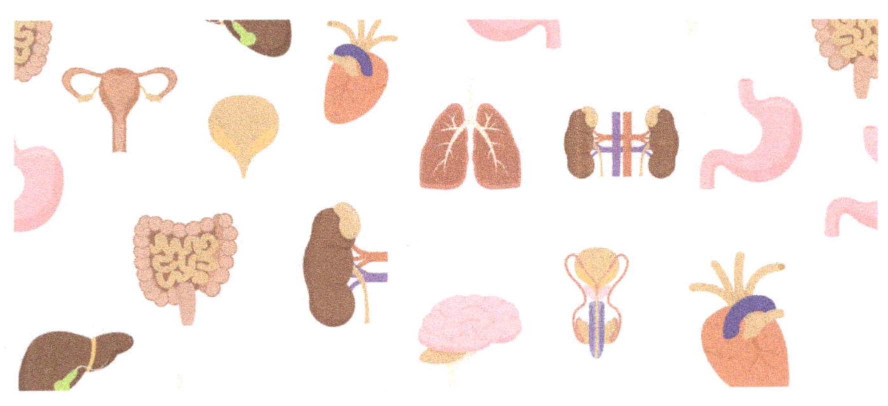

86. What does the brain do?

Answer: The brain controls everything we think, feel, and do.

87. How big is the brain?

Answer: It's about the size of two clenched fists.

88. What are nerves?

Answer: Nerves are like wires that carry messages between the brain and body.

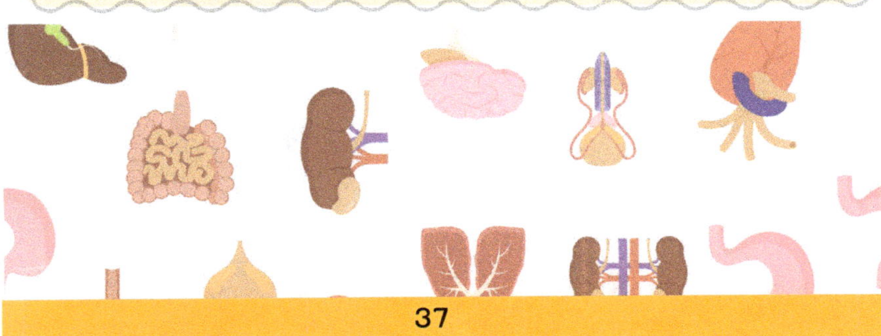

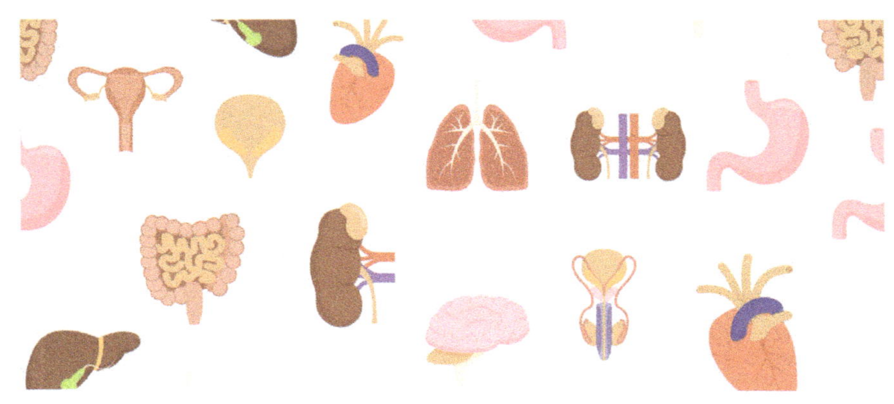

89. How does the brain send messages?

Answer: It sends messages through the nervous system using electrical signals.

90. What is the spinal cord?

Answer: The spinal cord is a long bundle of nerves that connects the brain to the rest of the body.

91. Why do we have reflexes?

Answer: Reflexes protect us by making us react quickly to danger.

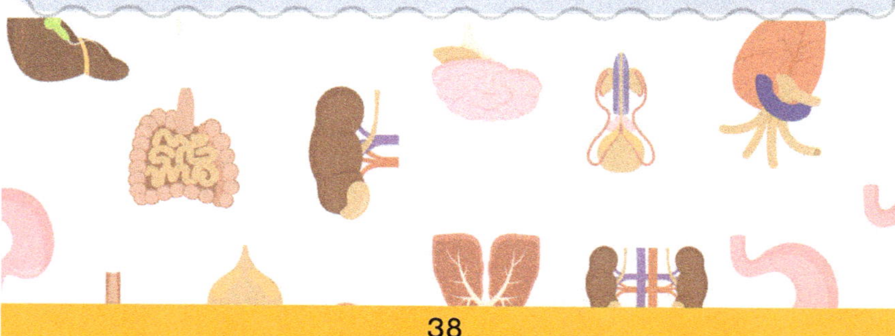

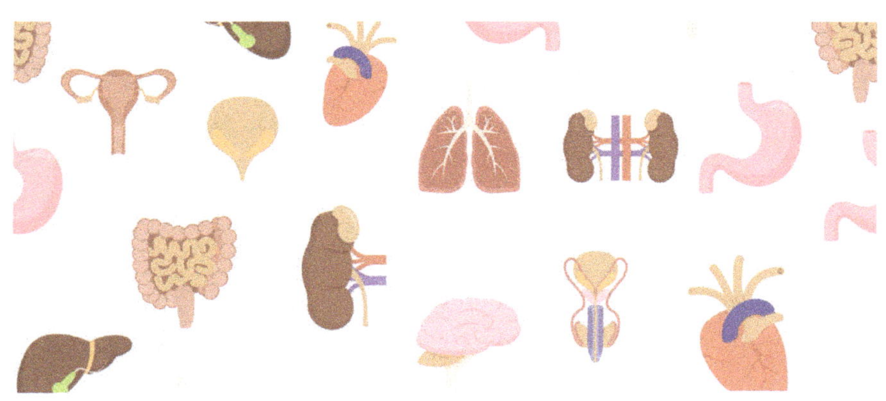

92. What is memory?

Answer: Memory is how the brain stores and remembers information.

93. Why do we dream?

Answer: Dreams happen when the brain processes thoughts and memories during sleep.

94. Why do we think??

Answer: Thinking helps us solve problems, make decisions, and learn new things.

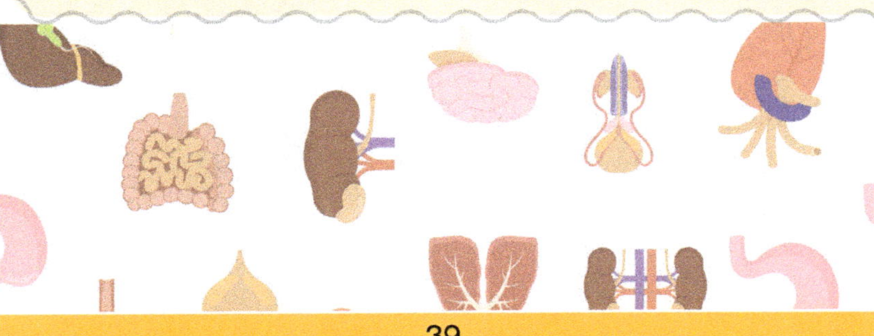

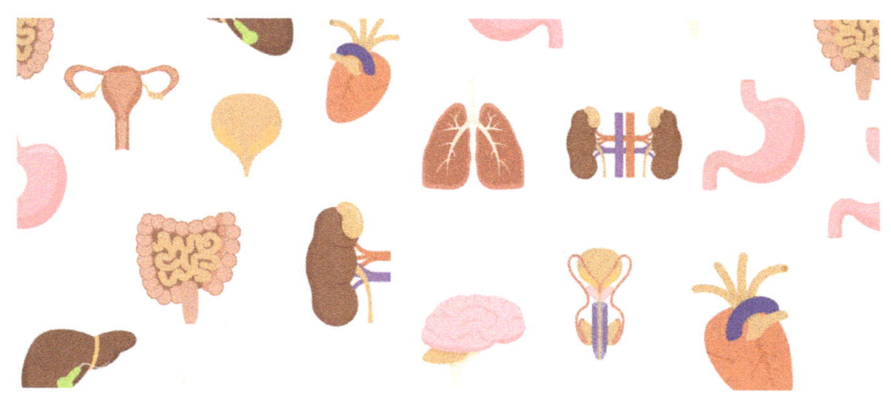

95. What is the cerebrum?

Answer: The cerebrum is the largest part of the brain, helping us think, learn, and move.

96. What is the cerebellum?

Answer: The cerebellum helps with balance and coordination.

97. Why do we need sleep?

Answer: Sleep lets our brain and body rest and recharge.

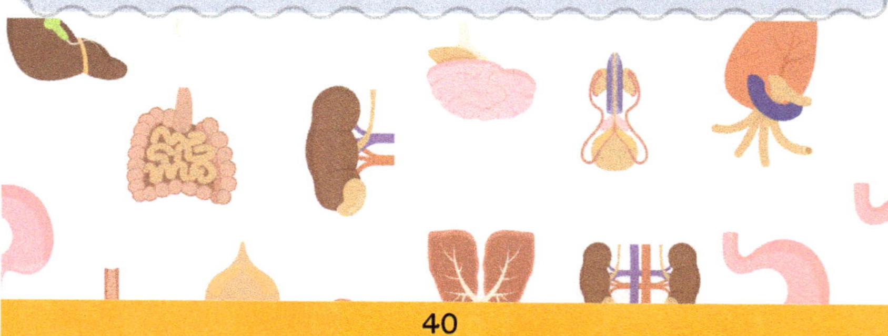

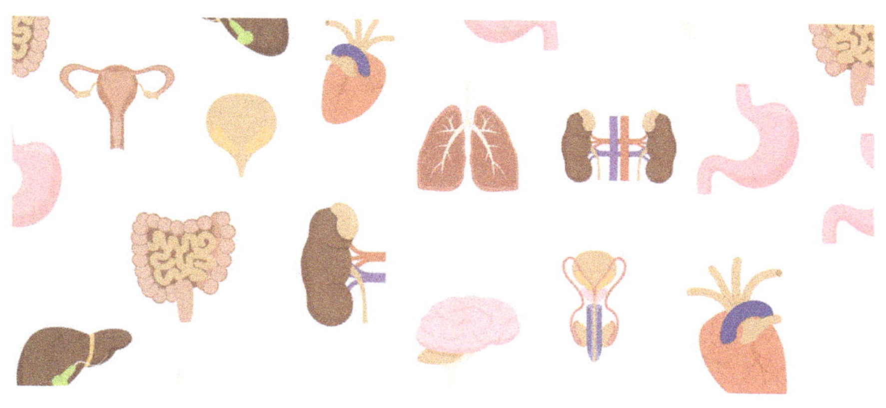

98. How fast can the brain send signals?

Answer: Brain signals can travel as fast as 250 miles per hour!

99. What is the brain made of?

Answer: The brain is made of neurons, blood vessels, and supportive tissues.

100. Why do we get headaches?

Answer: Headaches can be caused by stress, dehydration, or tiredness.

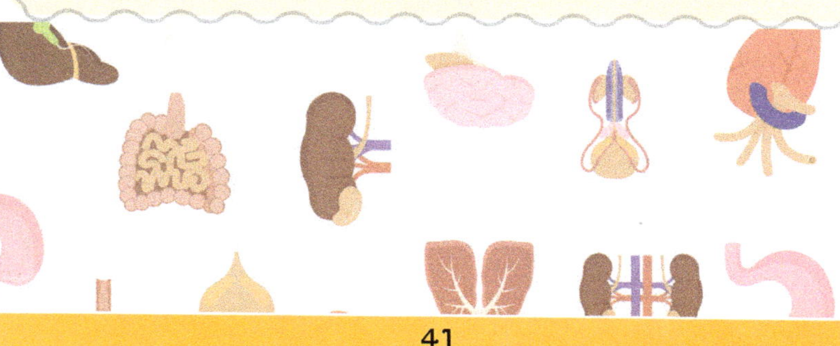

Senses

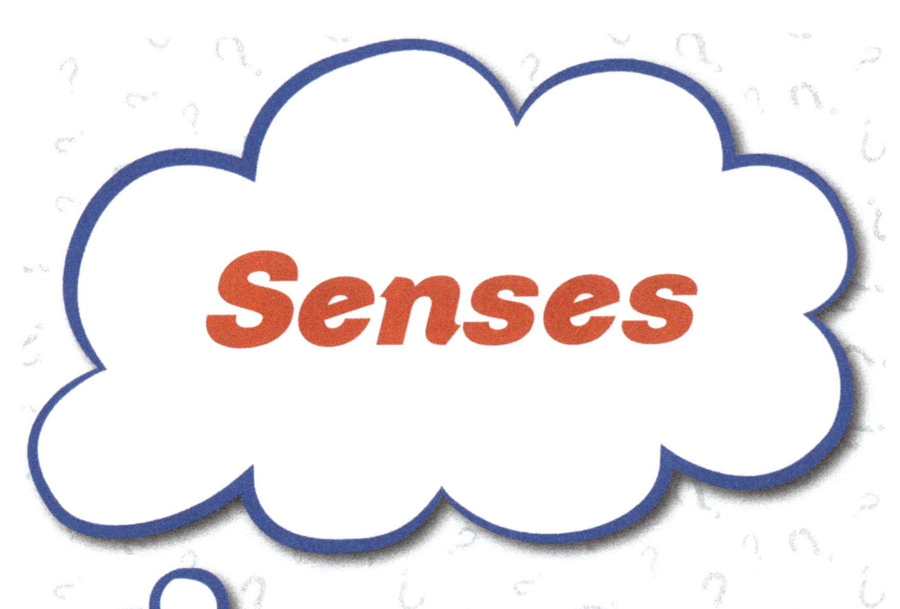

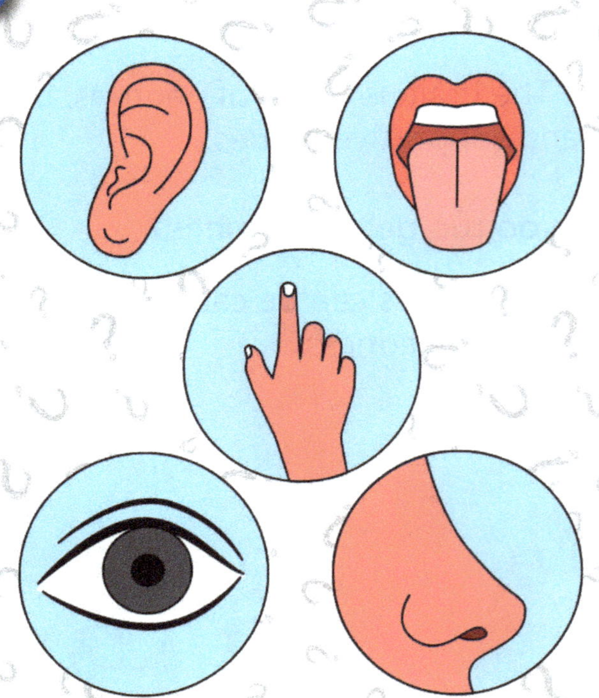

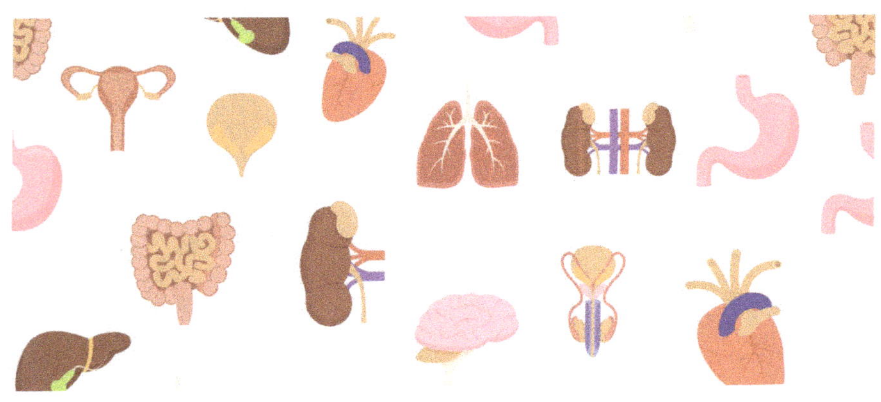

101. What are the five senses?

Answer: Sight, hearing, smell, taste, and touch.

102. How do we see?

Answer: Our eyes take in light, which the brain turns into images.

103. Why do we blink?

Answer: Blinking keeps our eyes moist and protects them from dust.

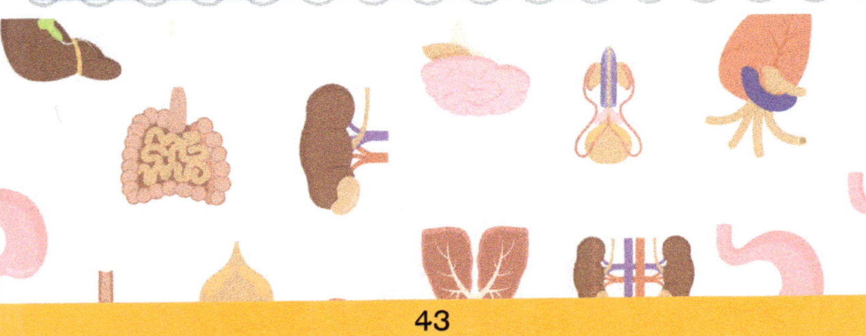

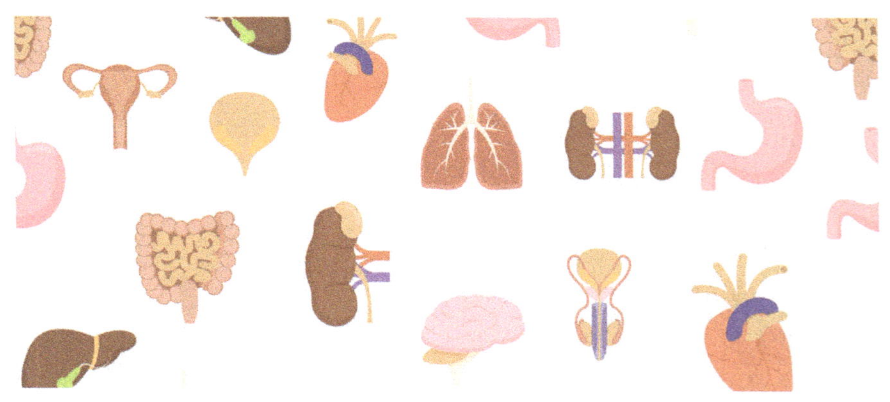

104. Why do we cry?

Answer: Crying helps clean our eyes and release emotions.

105. How do we hear?

Answer: Sound waves travel into our ears, and the brain turns them into sounds.

106. What is an eardrum?

Answer: The eardrum is a thin piece of skin that vibrates when sound hits it.

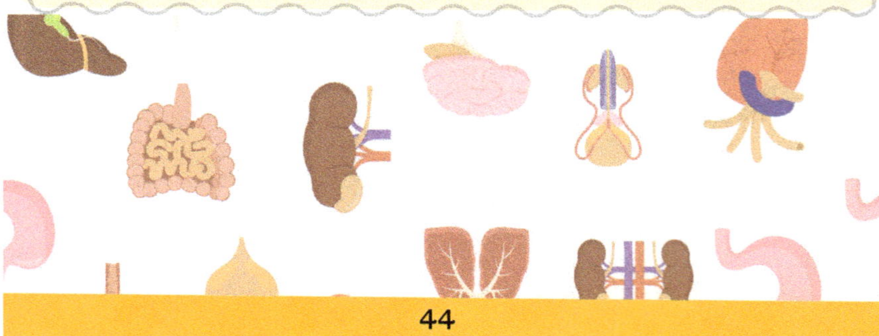

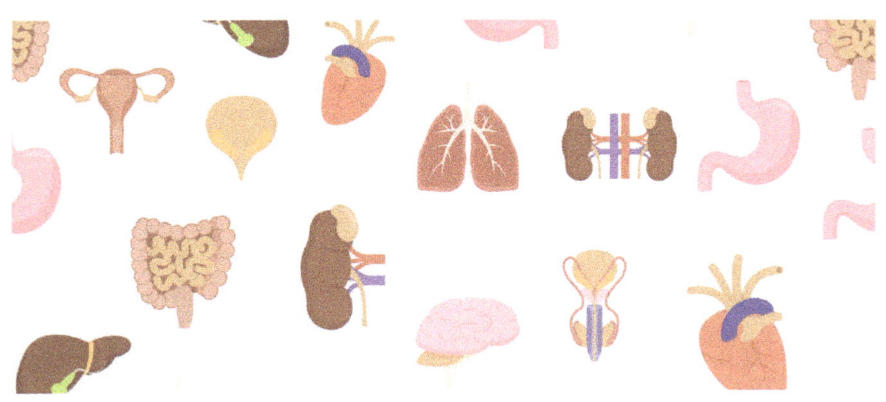

107. Why do we have two ears?

Answer: Two ears help us figure out where sounds are coming from.

108. How do we smell things?

Answer: Our nose detects smells, and the brain identifies them.

109. What are taste buds?

Answer: Taste buds are tiny bumps on the tongue that detect flavors.

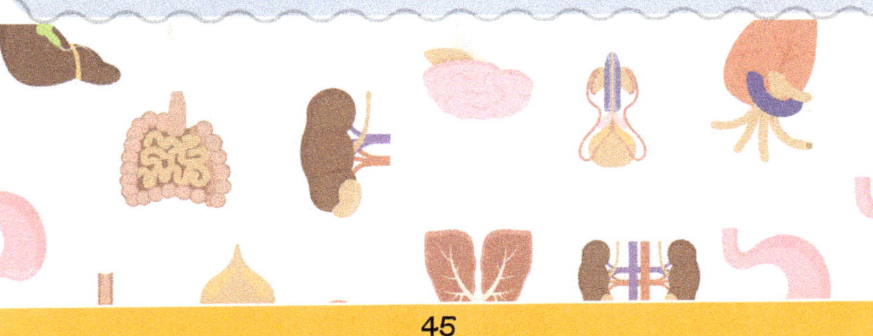

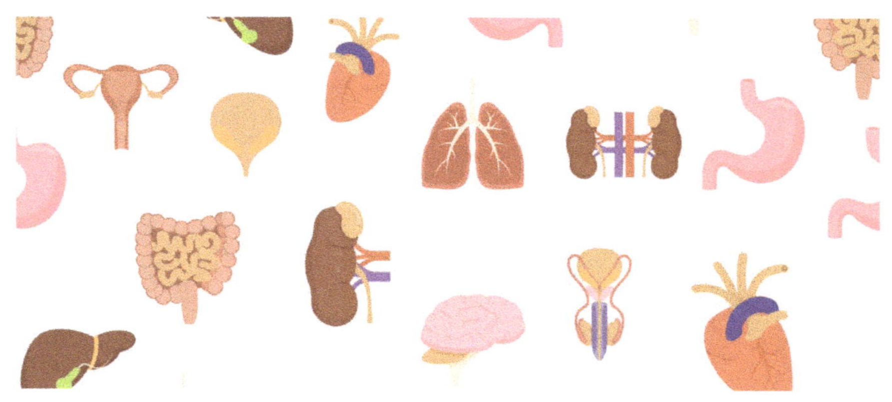

110. Why does food taste better when we're hungry?

Answer: Hunger makes our senses of taste and smell stronger.

111. How do we feel things?

Answer: Nerve endings in our skin send signals to the brain about what we touch.

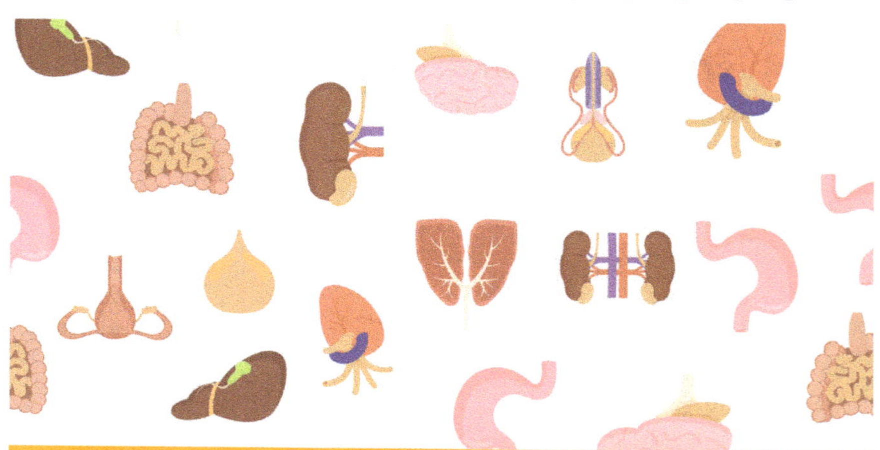

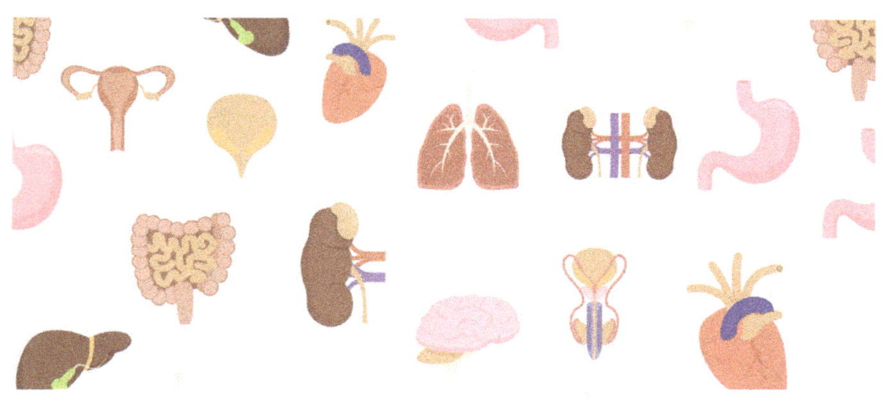

112. Why do we get ticklish?

Answer: Tickling triggers sensitive nerves in the skin.

113. Why do we get dizzy?

Answer: Dizziness happens when the balance system in our inner ear is confused.

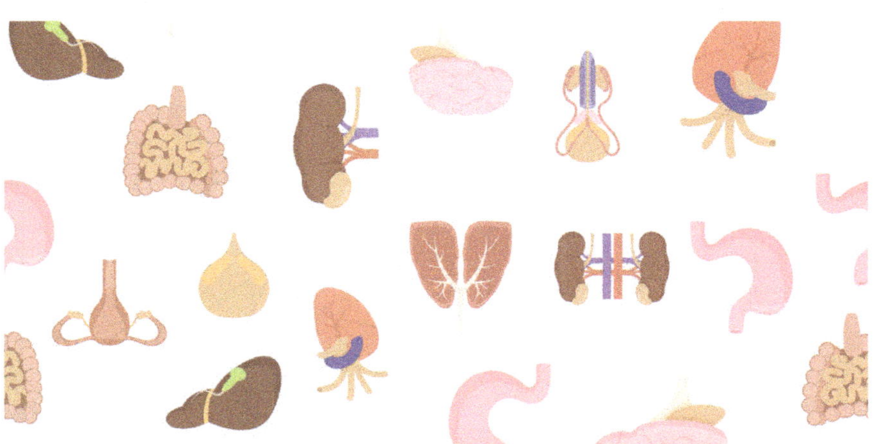

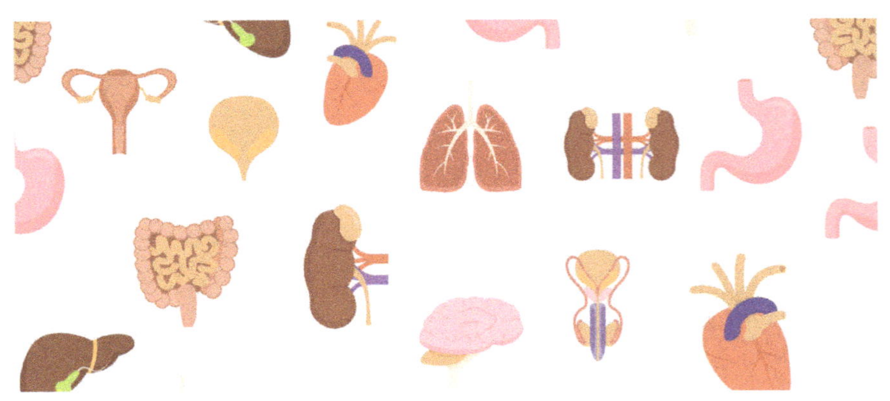

114. What is peripheral vision?

Answer: It's what we can see at the sides without turning our heads.

115. Why can't we see in the dark?

Answer: Our eyes need light to see, and there isn't enough light in the dark.

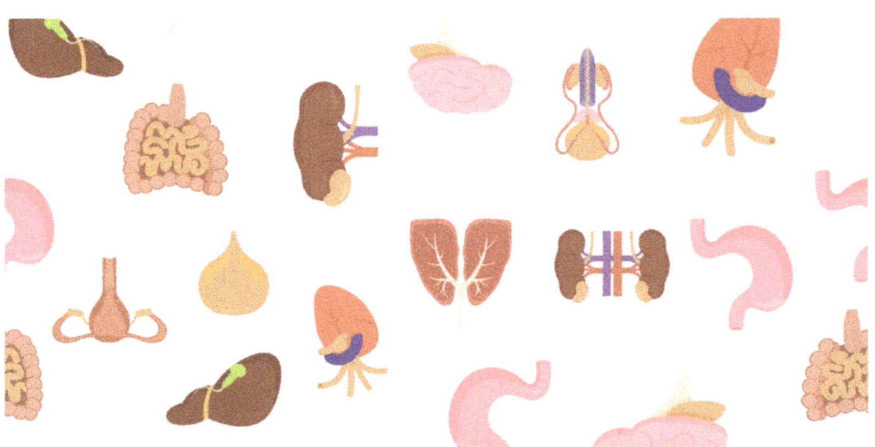

Weird and Fun Body Facts

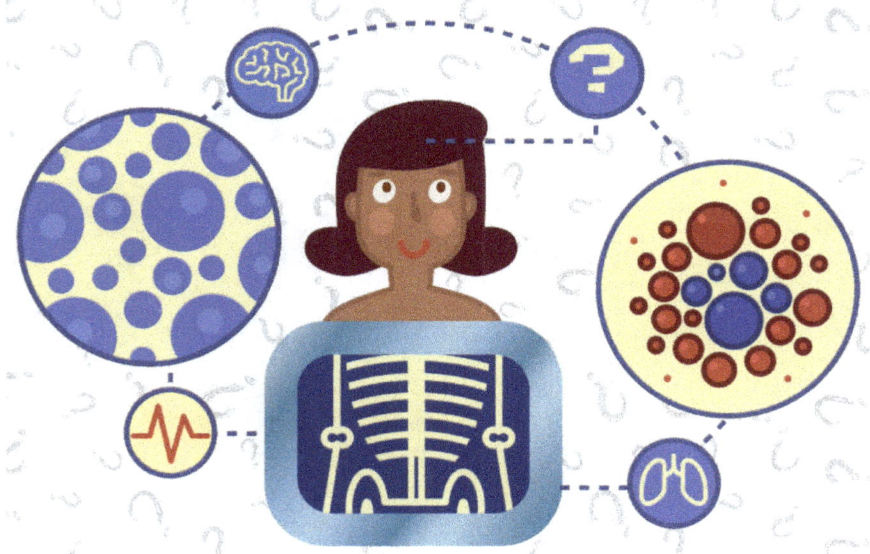

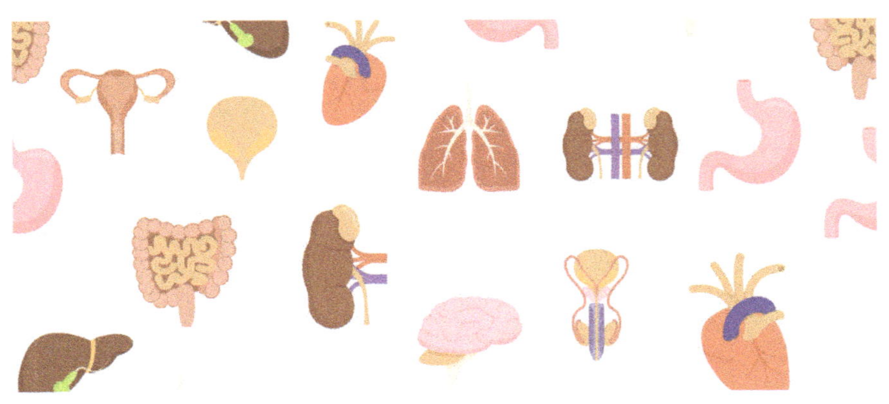

116. Why do we laugh?

Answer: Laughing is our body's way of showing happiness and connecting with others.

117. Why do we hiccup?

Answer: Hiccups happen when the diaphragm muscle suddenly tightens.

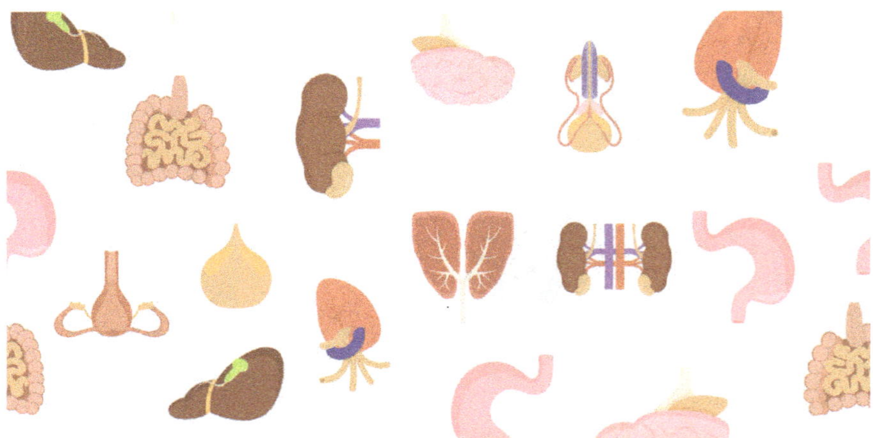

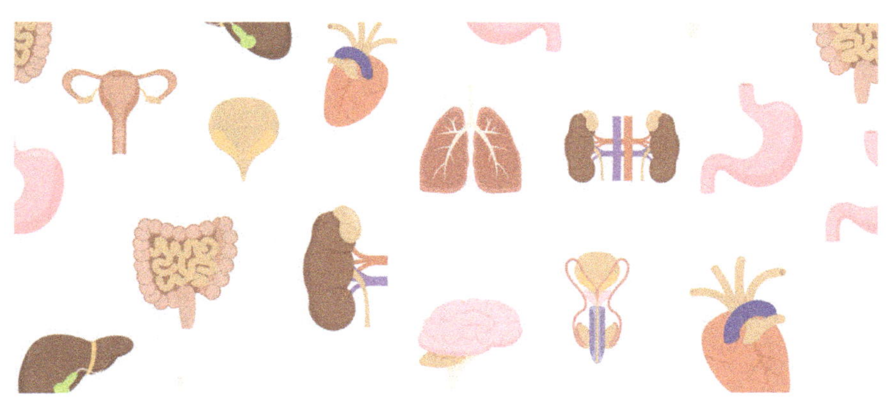

118. Why do we burp?

Answer: Burping lets out extra air from the stomach.

119. Why do we get goosebumps?

Answer: Goosebumps help keep us warm by making hair stand up.

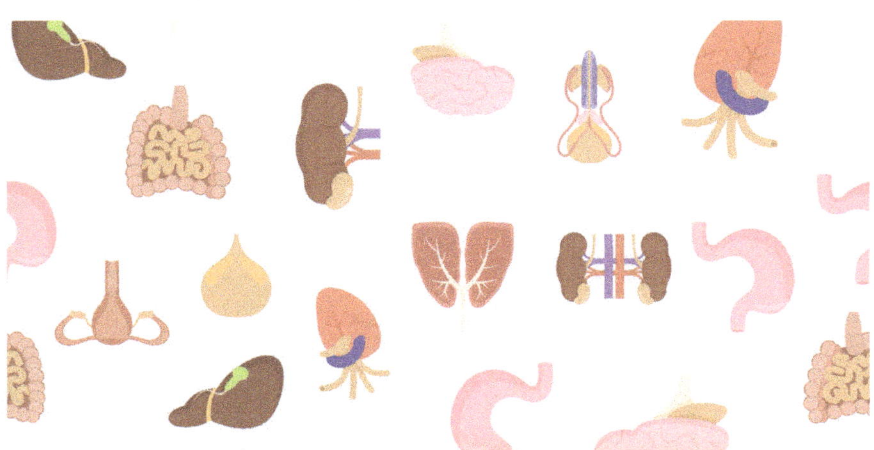

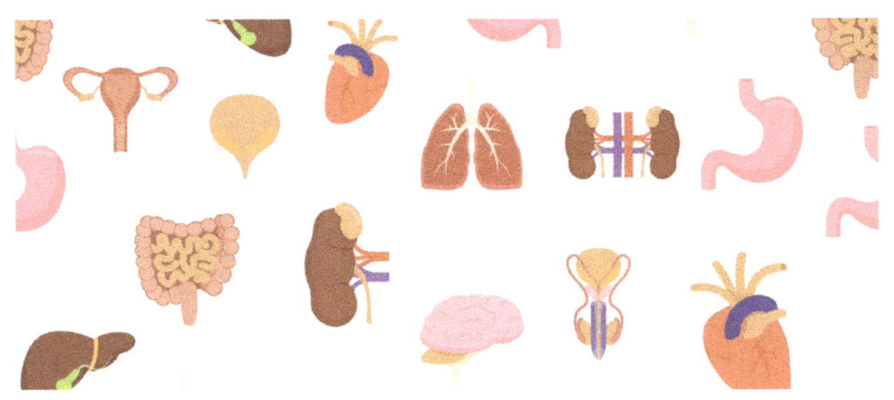

120. Why does our voice sound different when recorded?

Answer: We hear our voice differently through vibrations in our head.

121. Why do we snore?

Answer: Snoring happens when air has trouble moving through the throat while sleeping.

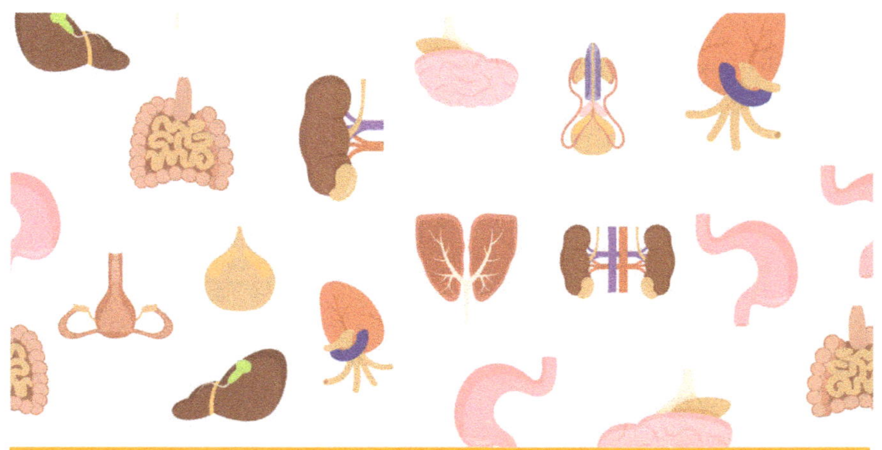

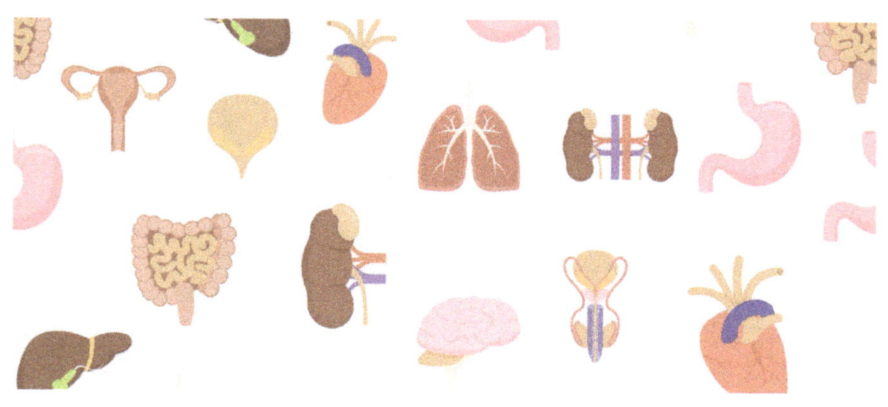

122. What is earwax?

Answer: Earwax is a sticky substance that protects ears from dirt and germs.

123. Why do our stomachs growl?

Answer: They growl when muscles move food or gas through the digestive system.

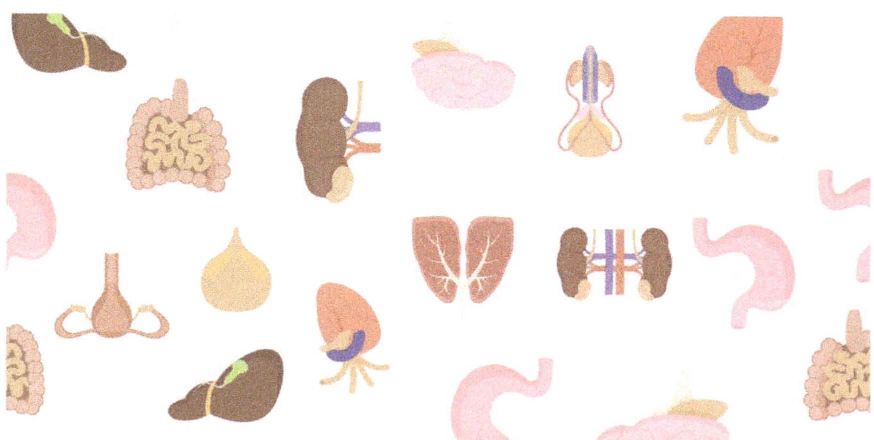

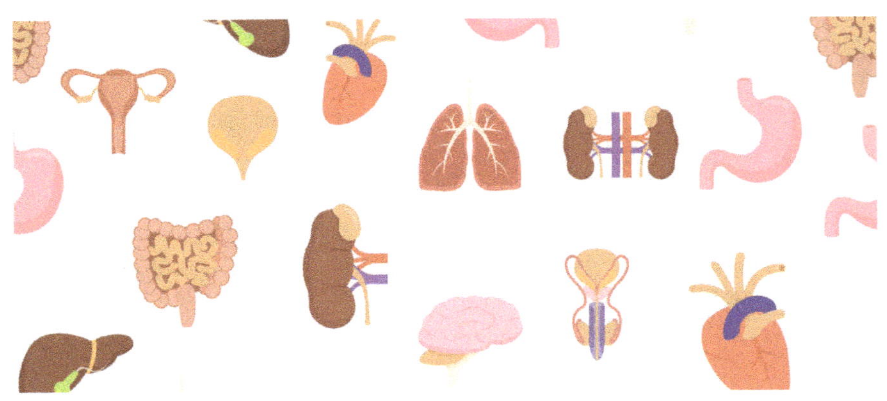

124. Why do we get tired?

Answer: Our body needs rest when it runs out of energy.

125. Why do we blush?

Answer: Blushing happens when blood rushes to our face, usually when we're embarrassed.

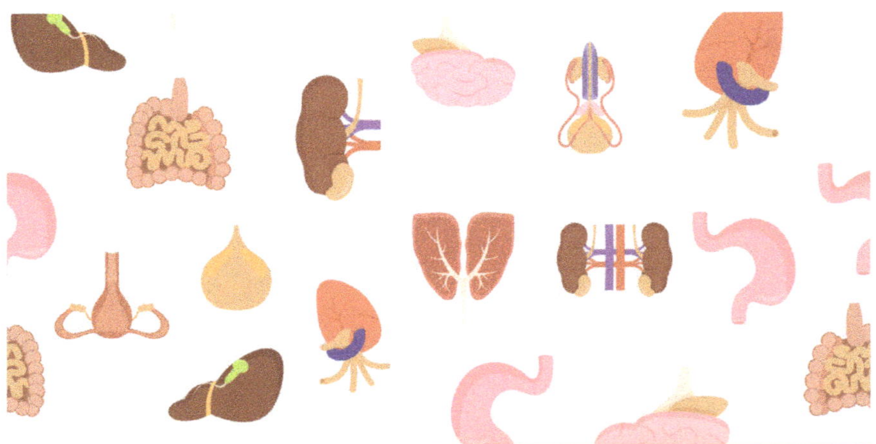

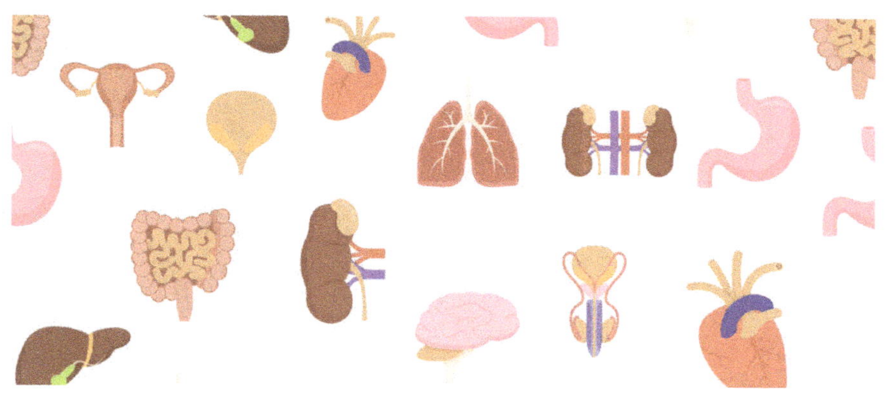

126. What are tonsils?

Answer: Tonsils are tissues at the back of the throat that help fight germs.

127. Why do we yawn when others do?

Answer: Yawning might be contagious because of social bonding or empathy.

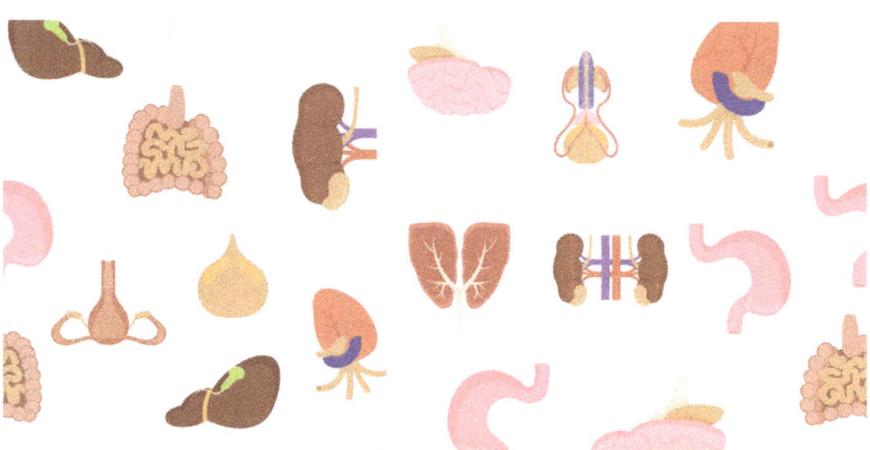

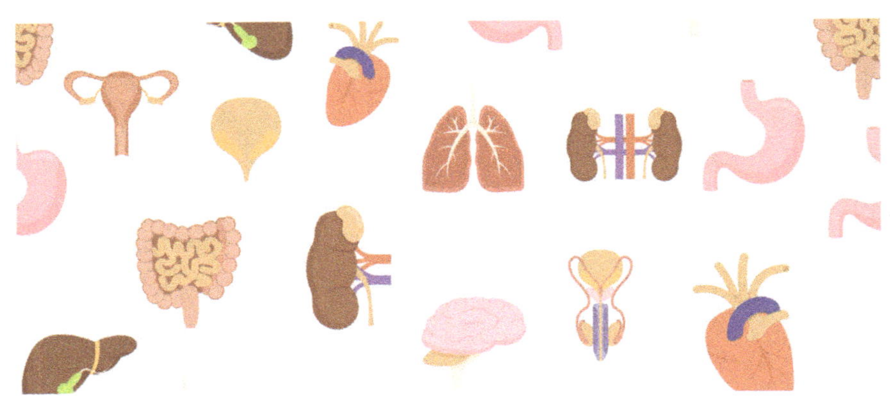

128. Why do we stretch when we wake up?

Answer: Stretching wakes up muscles and helps improve blood flow.

129. Why do we need two kidneys?

Answer: Two kidneys clean our blood and remove waste from the body.

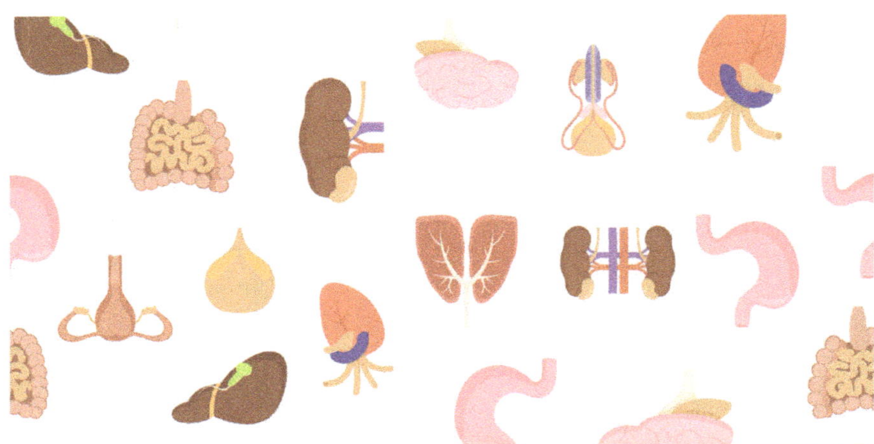

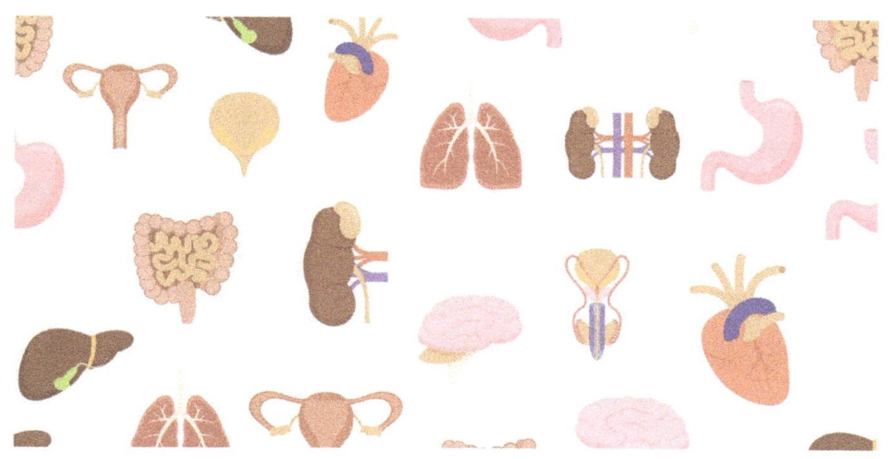

130. What is the appendix?

Answer: The appendix is a small, tube-like organ that doesn't have a clear function.

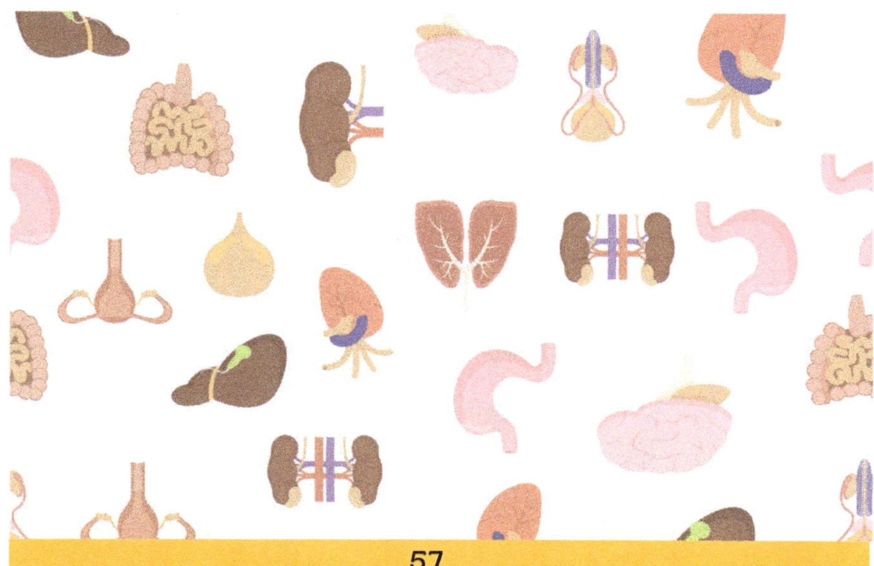

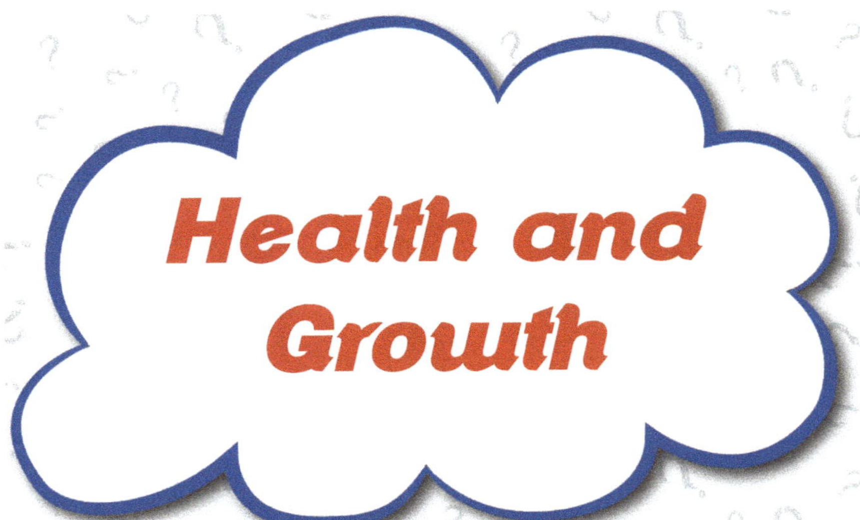

Health and
Growth

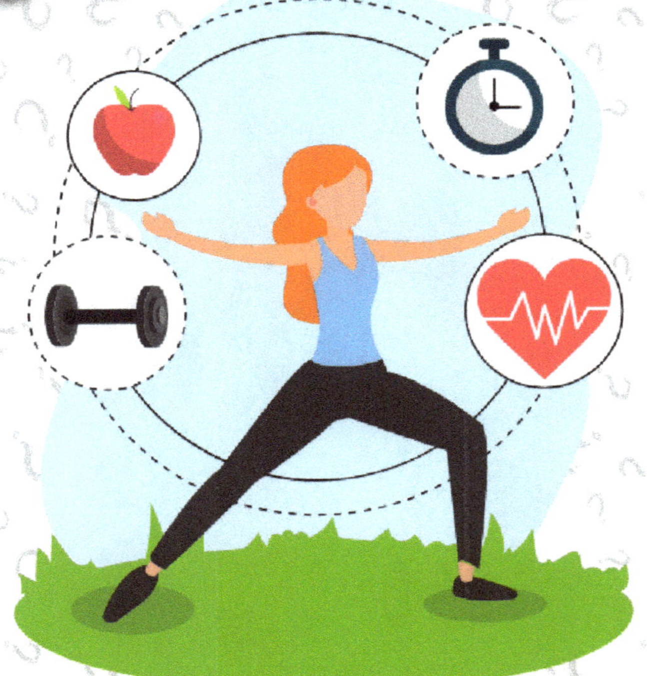

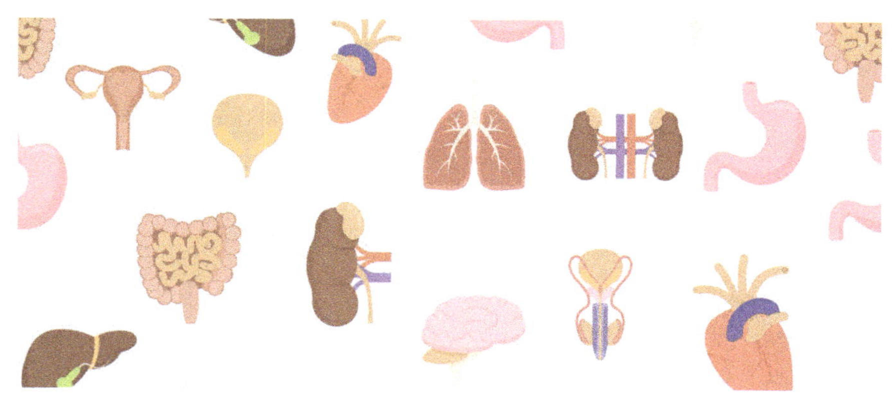

131. Why do we need to exercise?

Answer: Exercise keeps our body strong and healthy.

132. Why do we need to drink water?

Answer: Water keeps us hydrated and helps all our organs work.

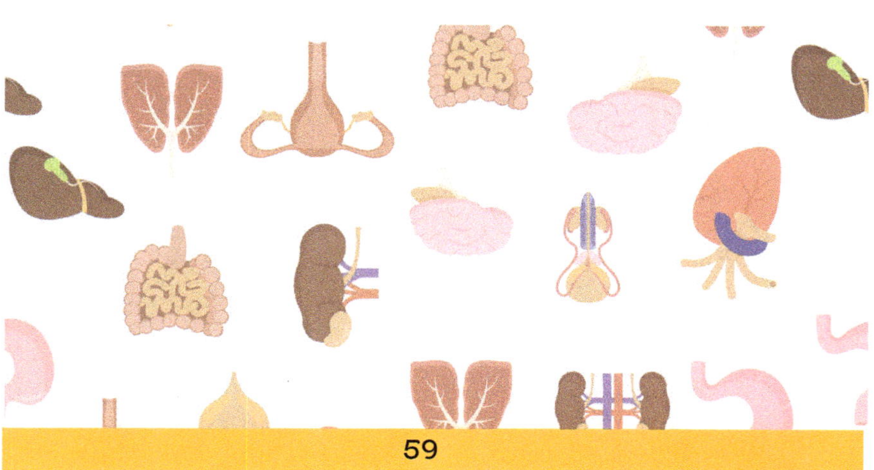

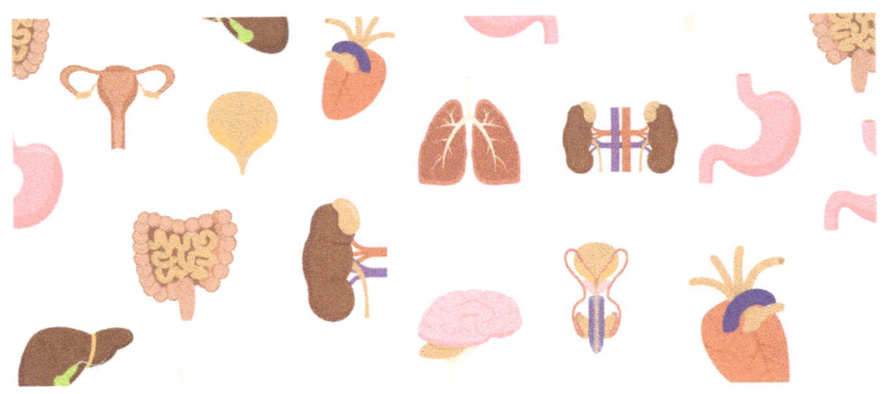

133. Why do we need vitamins?

Answer: Vitamins keep our body healthy and help it grow.

134. Why do we sleep?

Answer: Sleep lets our brain and body rest and repair.

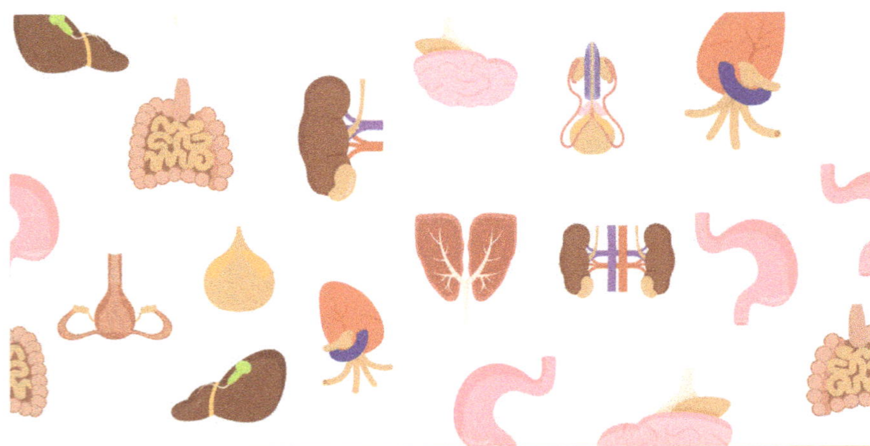

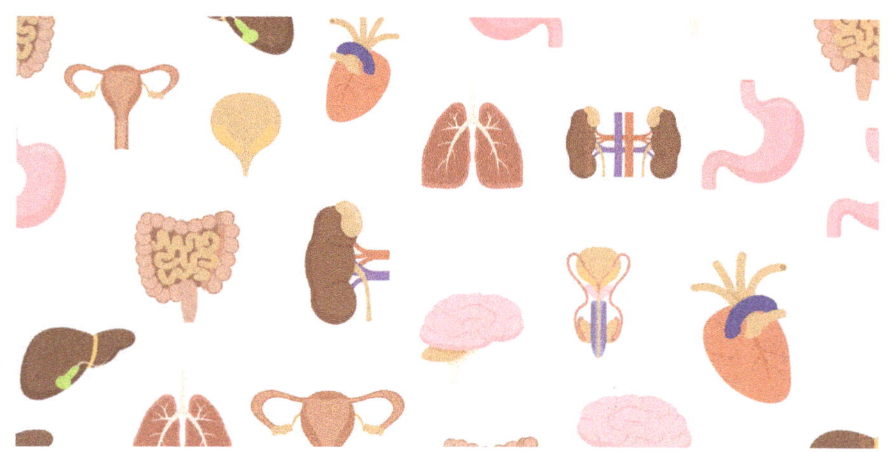

135. Why do we need to brush our teeth?

Answer: Brushing removes germs and prevents cavities.

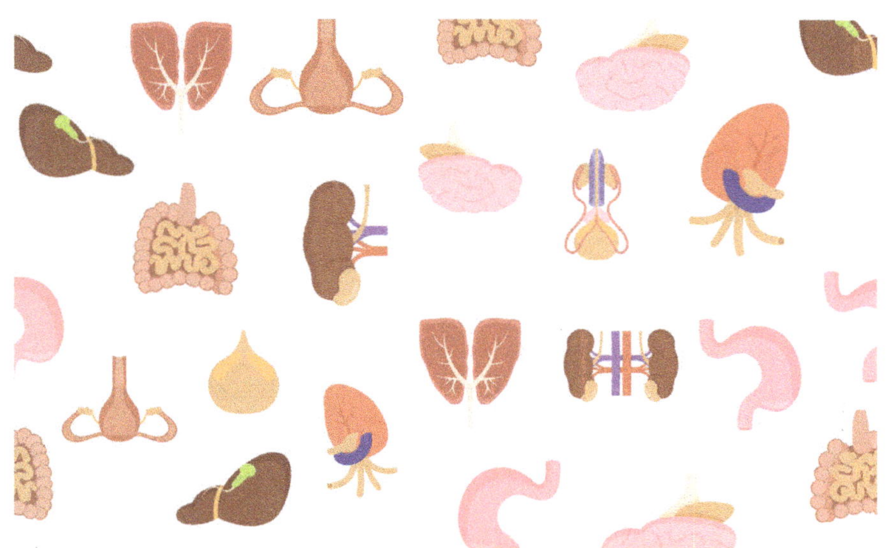

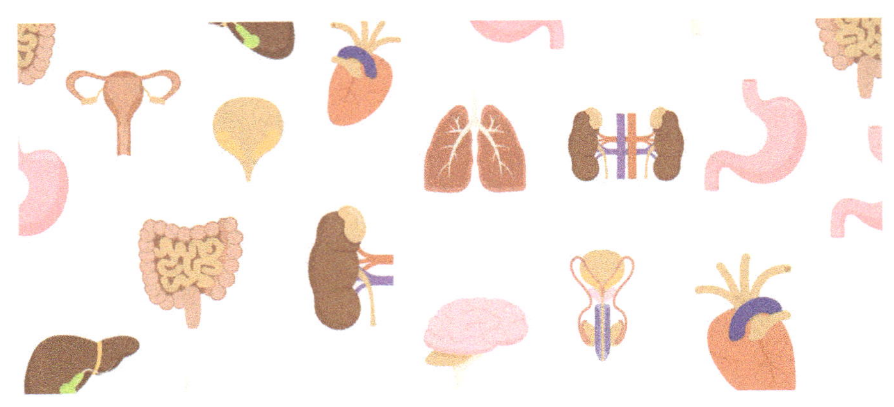

136. Why do we get sick?

Answer: Germs like bacteria and viruses can make us sick.

137. What is a fever?

Answer: A fever is the body's way of fighting germs.

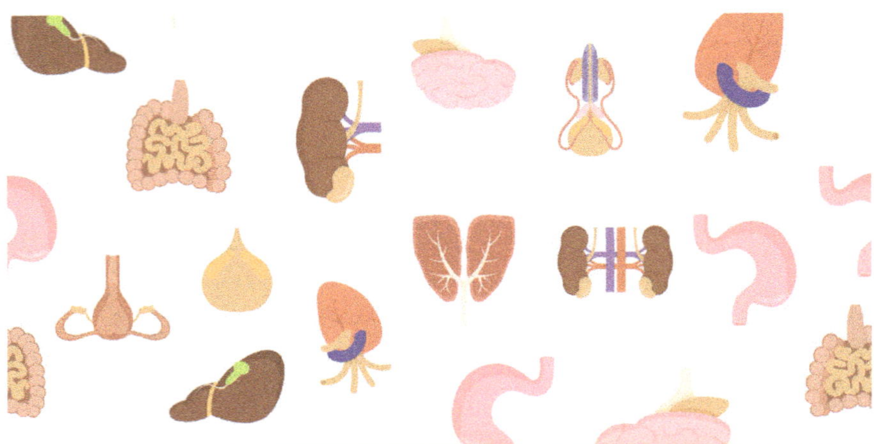

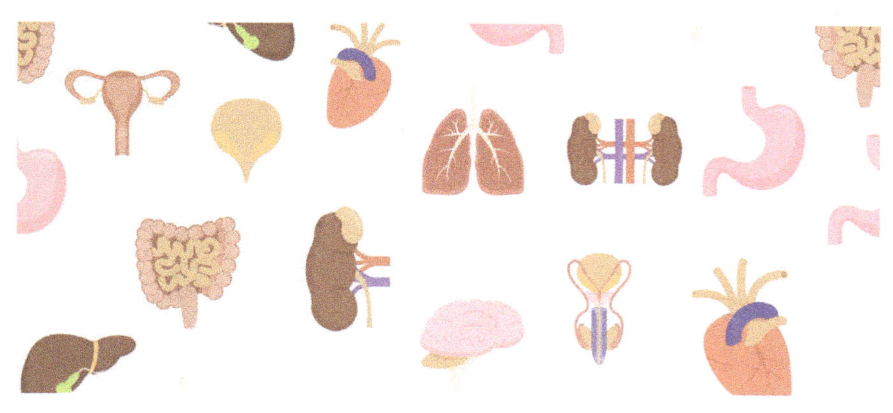

138. Why do we take medicine?

Answer: Medicine helps the body heal and fight illnesses.

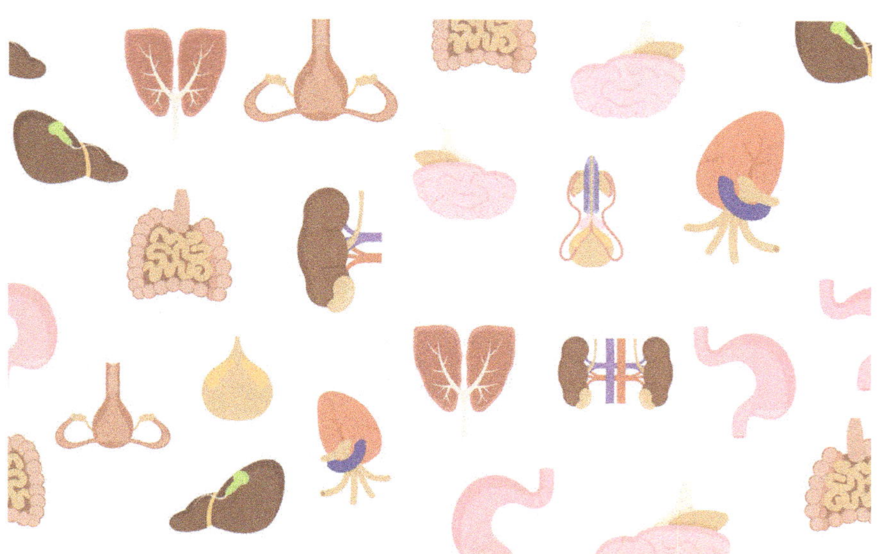

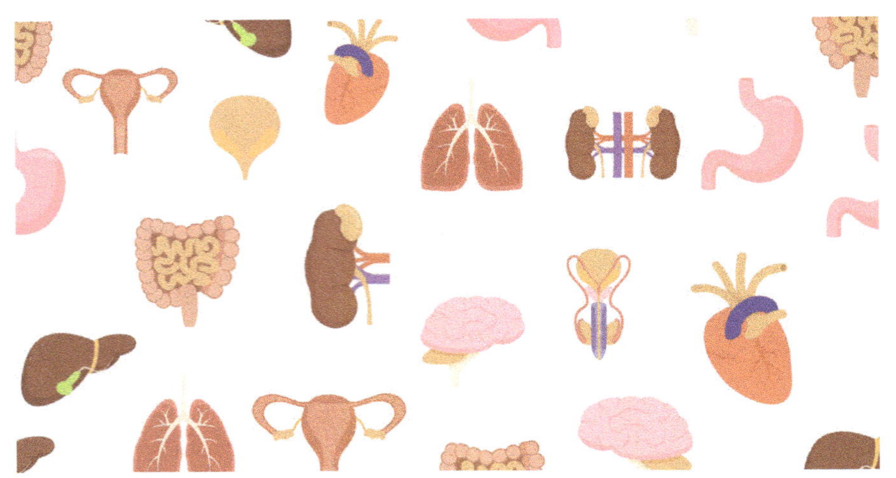

139. How does the body heal cuts?

Answer: Blood forms a scab to protect the wound while new skin grows.

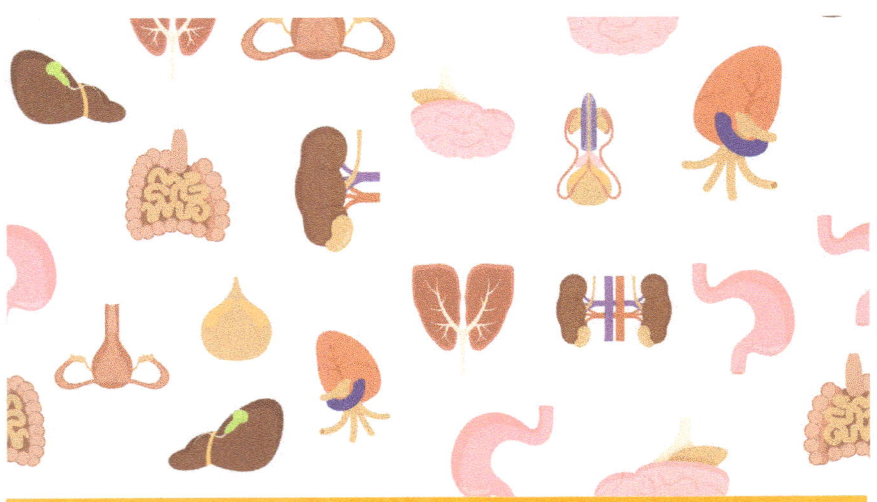

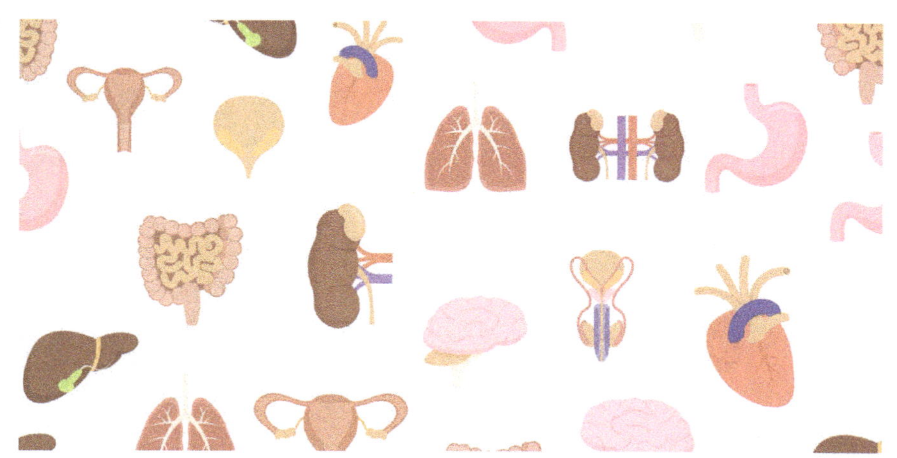

140. Why do we get shots?

Answer: Shots help prevent diseases by boosting the immune system.

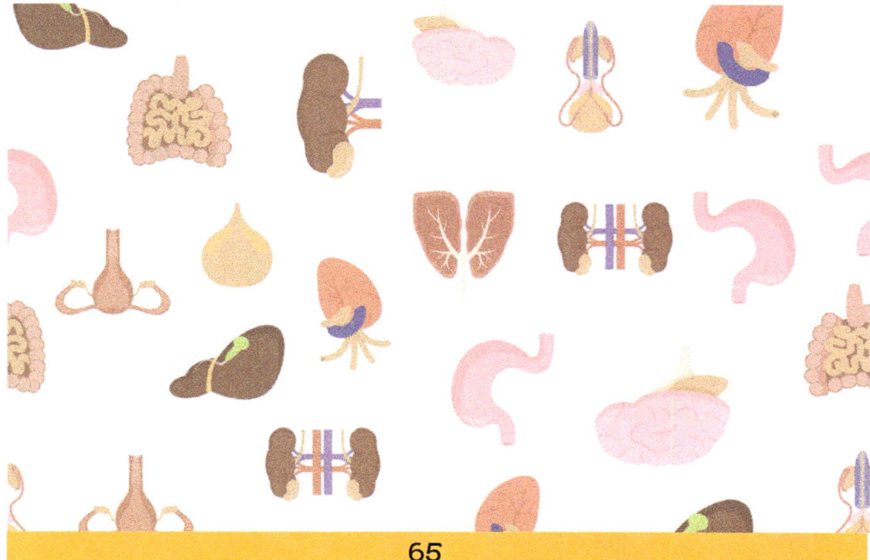

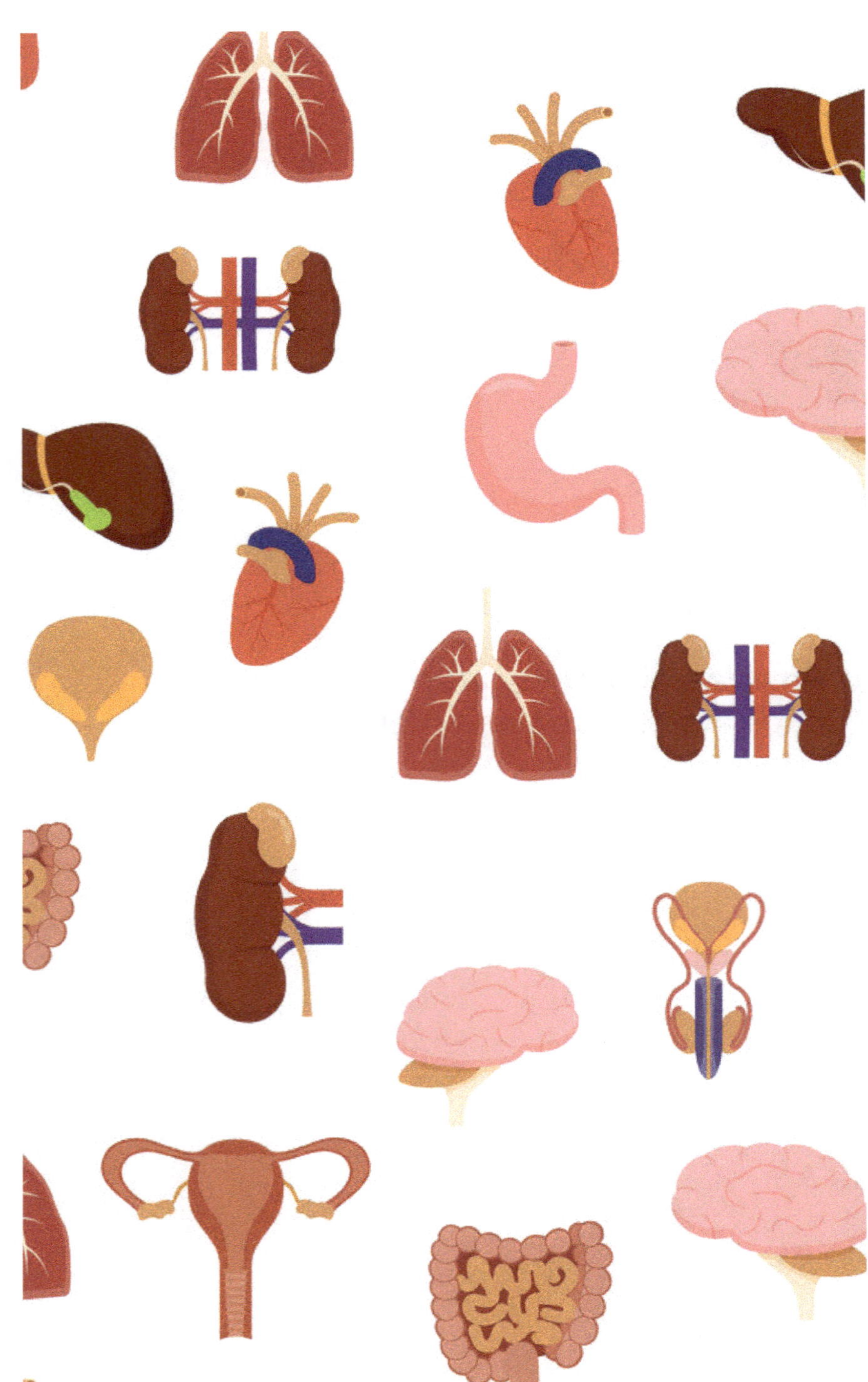